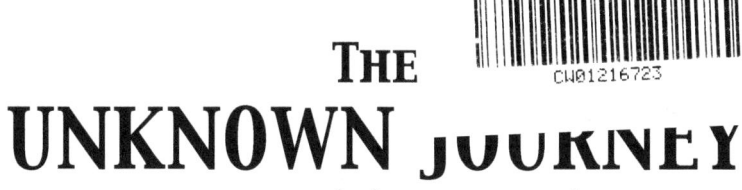

THE UNKNOWN JOURNEY
Surviving Hodgkin's Lymphoma

By
JOSEPH ANAMAN

Pegasus Publishing

Pegasus Publishing

P.O. Box 980, Edgecliff
NSW, Australia, 2027
www: linkageinc.co
Email: pegasuspublishing@iinet.net.au

First published in Australia by Pegasus Publishing in 2016

Copyright © Joseph Anaman 2016

All rights reserved. This book or any portion thereof may not be reproduced or used in any manner whatsoever without the express written permission of the publisher except for the use of brief quotations in a book review. If any part of this publication infringes on your copyright in any way, please contact the publisher.

National Library of Australia
Cataloguing-in-Publication Entry
THE UNKNOWN JOURNEY: Surviving Hodgkin's Lymphoma
Anaman, Joseph, 1967

Subjects:
Cancer, Hodgkin's Lymphoma, Lymphoma, Spirituality, Christianity, Christian Faith, Human Life, Survival.

ISBN: 978-0-9942014-9-2

Book layout and design by Pegasus Publishing

Front Cover:
'Sunset at Azul Fives' (1/10/2011) by Charlie Stinchcombe. Available at
https://www.flickr.com/photos/47000103@N05/6334538750
under a Creative Commons Attribution 2.0 Generic License. Full terms at
http://creativecommons.org/licenses/by/2.0.

Also available in eBook format [ISBN 978-0-9942014-8-5]

Printed and bound in Australia by IngramSpark.

JOSEPH ANAMAN

Pegasus Publishing • Sydney

"An honest, raw account of an unimaginable health battle that is written in an entertaining and thought provoking fashion, which will surely inspire you."
Moritz Schreiber

"Epic… a bittersweet and moving account that lingers in the mind."
Fred Nelson

"In this magnificent, deeply moving account, the struggles of Joseph Anaman illuminate the ways, against all odds, that people can overcome devastation and adversity."
Ross Sinclair

"A vastly entertaining feat, written throughout a desperate personal struggle."
Joan Matlin

"Joseph provides an unpatronising, brutally honest and frequently humorous roller coaster ride, of the life of someone battling with cancer. An essential read for patients, family and carers."
Dr. Michael Anaman

Dedication

I dedicate this book to anyone suffering hardship in their life, but especially to my wonderful Mum, who after being a part of me for the last 48 years, passed away in October 2015.

All we need is Love!

Foreword

I have had the great pleasure of looking after Joseph Anaman for the last five years since he developed Nodular Lymphocyte-Predominant Hodgkin Lymphoma.

Nodular lymphocyte-predominant Hodgkin Lymphoma is a rare subtype of a Hodgkin lymphoma. Hodgkin Lymphoma accounts for less than 1% of all cancers in Australia and only 5-10% of these are the Nodular Lymphocyte Predominant subtype. It typically affects males aged from 30-50 and is slow-growing and responsive to chemotherapy and radiotherapy, but with a tendency to relapse and to transform into a more aggressive lymphoma, unlike the more common forms of Hodgkin Lymphoma.

Because of the small numbers of patients around the world, the ideal treatments are still not certain, but the disease has been shown to respond well to anti-CD20 antibody therapy. Most patients with this lymphoma have a good long-term survival and the object is to treat the disease with the aim of reducing relapse and treatment-related toxicity.

Joseph is in many ways a typical patient with this lymphoma, being a man aged 30-50 years old and having experienced a relapse in his condition, but he has been unfortunate to have had short remissions lasting around two years and some treatment-related toxicity. He has been very brave and open about his lymphoma and I'm amazed and delighted that he has been able to put together this book in between work, family and a very demanding treatment schedule.

Dr. Susan MacCallum
MBBS (Hons 1) FRACP FRCPA

Preface

Life is full of surprises, each with its own twists and turns for everyone to experience in their own way. Then, out of the blue, a day may arrive when you are faced with a life threatening decision. What do you do and how do you respond?

When you hear the word cancer, what goes through your mind? Do you know of any friends or family who have had it? If so, how did you help them and what do you say and do to make them feel better? It isn't easy for the sufferer or for their close family and friends.

I travelled this journey and more often than not kept a journal on a day-to-day basis, recording what I experienced while riding the ups and downs of undergoing chemotherapy and radiation. In taking you by the hand through my two-year battle with Hodgkin's Lymphoma, I hope the reader will gain an understanding of what it feels like to experience the physical and emotional roller-coaster ride of cancer sufferers.

With absolutely no control of what lies ahead, the journey is definitely a daunting experience. Even with loved ones to help you through, I feel that nowadays, in the midst of the age of technology, there is a general lack of information regarding how to deal with cancer from a mental, spiritual and emotional standpoint.

Therefore, I wrote this book to encourage all people suffering with Hodgkin's Lymphoma, cancer or other such debilitating problems. No matter what your circumstances may be, life is worth living. My hope is that readers gain an insight into how this experience changed my way of thinking and opened my mind, to seeing the world in a much more positive way.

Joseph Anaman

Contents

Chapter 1	Damned	9
Chapter 2	The Struggle Ahead	19
Chapter 3	Fighting Back	27
Chapter 4	The Grind	37
Chapter 5	Keeping Sane	44
Chapter 6	A Poison Chalice	54
Chapter 7	Descending	65
Chapter 8	Taking A Break	73
Chapter 9	Restless & Rocky	82
Chapter 10	Overwhelmed	90
Chapter 11	Faith & Love	97
Chapter 12	Glimmer of Hope	107
Chapter 13	Unreal Dreams	117
Chapter 14	That's Life	126
Thank You		135

CHAPTER 1

Damned

The Unknown

Yesterday I completely shaved my hair! But today, staring at the man in the mirror, I wondered what this face would look like in a few months' time? I don't really know why I did this. Even though my doctor told me it happens to fewer people nowadays, was I expecting my hair to fall out on day one? I normally wear a zero haircut so who would notice anyway? That night I woke up a couple of times, tossing and turning, wondering how I'd be feeling this time tomorrow, next week and whether I'd still be on this earth in a few months time.

We are not strictly religious folk, but my wife Jude and I prayed for a positive outcome, for great times ahead, for our families, for our friends, for our church members and for each and everyone who was suffering or going through trials of their own. We also prayed to encourage and strengthen others who might one day have to face their own daunting journeys.

On the way to the hospital, I was surprisingly calm. Was it because over the last few months my visits had been so numerous, you could almost call them routine? At times I thought it had come almost to the point where I felt I was on my way to work, but this time was different.

The check-in routine was the same every time. The personnel on the information desk would greet me with a friendly nod and a forced smile. As I walked past the department where blood testing was conducted, one of the staff would acknowledge me with a greeting. "Morning Joseph".

At which I would reply "Morning, how are you?"

I was relieved that they didn't want to strike up a conversation, especially today. In the real world, the reaction on peoples' faces said it all whenever I mentioned the 'c' word. 'C' being for chemotherapy and cancer. Their predictable expression would always be one of shock, surprise or immense sympathy. "Ohhh.... you poor thing", and "My Aunt Beryl went through that a few years ago", were very common types of responses.

I often felt compelled to ask that million-dollar question, expecting a million dollar response. "By the way, how is that member of your family going?" The common answer was usually a delayed one... and given in a rather hushed stutter.

"Ummmm.... she... umm... she passed away."

Well "that kind of reply really boosted my confidence no end... NOT!"... my inner-self would sarcastically whisper. You see, I didn't ever want to be fussed over, and the aftermath of a 'pity party' always left me feeling like an abandoned ship.

Family

My parents both came from Ghana formerly known as Gold Coast, which is situated in West Africa. My parents didn't inherit any of their country's riches as they both emigrated to the United Kingdom as qualified nurses. They wanted to make a better life for themselves and pioneer a new life, with their children being first generation English-born Africans. I have a younger brother Michael, and Sister Julia, and the three of us are very close. I also have another two half-brothers and two half-sisters who live in the United Kingdom and in Ghana.

Throughout the 1970's growing up in England wasn't at all easy. There was strong pressure from political parties opposed to immigrants taking jobs from the locals and so we, like many others suffered victimization, racial abuse and constant name calling from an early age, and especially throughout our school years. Despite that, we still made a lot of good friends along the way and developed thick skins to cope with the abuse. Now as adults we are much less sensitive and have a much greater awareness and acceptance of other cultures.

These days Britain is very multi-cultural and has come a long way in terms of social acceptance. This major cultural upheaval was probably due in part to two world wars, colonialization and a huge rise in immigration. The old country has also developed a dry sense of humour primarily caused by national sporting teams that don't really perform well on the world scene! Britain is fortunate also to have developed a culture of musicians, actors, entertainers and comedians together with their various regional accents (that no one in the world understands), which has contributed greatly to the acceptance of foreigners with a laugh here and there! Or, is it just due to the fact that England has crappy weather all year round?

In 1994, I ventured out on my own and emigrated from England to Australia to forge a new life by myself. Not long after I met my wonderful, loyal life partner and wife, Judy. Jude, as she prefers to be called, is two years younger than me, was born in New Zealand and is part Maori and part English due to her parents mixed heritage.

Jude is the eldest of four sisters but also has two elder brothers and two younger brothers. She works full time in retail and part time as a carer. Jude is an amazing woman and is very passionate about the welfare of people as she always jumps in to help others in their time of need. Our relationship is one of trust and respect for each other without stepping over each other's boundaries.

Together we are a blend of African and Maori cultures and our traditions revolve around large families, friends and friends of friends. Jude's two sons, Jesse aged 26 and Shannon aged 24, live together and have a close relationship, almost sharing the same group of friends.

Tahlia is our beautiful daughter at 16 years of age and lives at home with Jude and myself. She likes to hang out with us on holidays and when we eat out, whilst maintaining a healthy social calendar with her own friends.

We live in Malabar, which is still largely untouched by development, and by that I mean you can always find a car space next to the beach, without driving around endlessly in circles. There are no parking meters, so parking is easy and there are a number of up-market cafes and shops with very friendly and welcoming staff.

If you asked anyone who knows Malabar, they'd describe it as a low-density, friendly coastal community with a small beach and barbecue area. There are a couple of parks, which are occupied by dogs and their owners in the morning. When you pass people in the street you get a friendly greeting, or a smile is exchanged.

Diagnosis

The first time I came into contact with cancer, was back in 2010. I can clearly remember it was a stormy winters night, and I'd felt very ill all day. I just thought it was some bad food I'd eaten, but happened to catch sight of some blood that I eventually threw up. This was a concern, a grave concern as its not normal to vomit blood.

The next morning I immediately booked an appointment to see my local doctor and explained what had happened. He took a blood sample and told me he would send it to the pathology lab and I would receive the results within a few days.

Later that evening, while in my local supermarket shopping, I surprisingly received a phone call from my doctor in person, which was definitely abnormal and much sooner than I'd expected. He informed me that my blood test results came back very quickly and that a person's normal blood platelet count should be between 40,000 to 150,000 platelets per microliter of blood. However, my reading was just 20,000. This figure was just 'double dutch' to me of course, as I wasn't at all familiar with medical jargon or blood counts. I thought to myself...."maybe if I had a job as a Vampire I'd be able to shed some light on the matter!" ...not sunlight, though, as that would really do me in! Haha!

But my doctor jolted me out of that jovial thought and went on to say that I had better book myself in at the local hospital soon. He would, of course, fax them a letter of explanation. This all sounded a bit serious I thought, so when I arrived home I told my wife Jude what had happened. Straight away she flew into response mode, I could read the panic on her face and she insisted I get a move on with it.

After dinner, we went directly to the hospital. Both of us were surprised at how efficient the hospital staff were when I told the receptionist my name. I was immediately whisked off to the Intensive Care Unit where I stayed for the next three days and nights. I had a raft of blood tests, a number of urine analyses and was subjected to a lot of repetitive questions regarding symptoms I had or hadn't experienced, each and every time medical staff entered my room.

It was during this time that I was informed I had developed an auto-immune disorder, which was attacking my body and destroying healthy body cells, which in extreme cases can result in internal bleeding. Also, if I managed to cut myself whilst my blood platelets were this low, uncontrolled bleeding would occur and be very difficult to stop.

On the fourth day, medication was issued for me to take home to help adjust my blood platelets. However, because of the nature of my job as a chef, I wasn't allowed to go to work, which I didn't mind for one moment. I was not in any discomfort at this stage, in fact I actually convinced myself that all the symptoms I was experiencing were just related to job stress, brought on by my increasingly difficult work situation.

Whilst the fractious work situation continued an appointment had been arranged for me with a haematologist, a specialist doctor who studies and treats blood conditions and disorders. Dr. Susan MacCallum or, Dr. Susan as I came to know her is a middle-aged medical specialist with a wealth of knowledge accompanied by a warm and very understanding smile. After just 15 minutes with her I understood a whole lot more about blood platelets. She told me exactly what situation I was in and how quickly we had to move to combat the problem. She also stressed how critical it was for me not to be in contact with any sharp objects, especially in my industry, just in case I was cut and the bleeding became hard to stop.

She told me of a window fitter who had low blood platelets for quite a few months. I asked what happened to him, but the reply was short and sweet. He had to quit his job! Her advice for me was to take a few weeks off work until my platelets were at a higher count, so she wrote me a medical certificate. At this stage I wasn't too concerned about the seriousness of the medical condition I was now facing, but more about my future work situation in the kitchen.

After a further nine months of what became torture at work and constantly walking on egg shells, the penny finally dropped! Having often discussed the situation with Jude and after seeking advice through Legal Aid, I came to a conclusion. Even though my wage was good, the working hours were great and no weekends were required, it became obvious that it was time to leave my extremely stressful job. After much soul-searching, I realised that life was just too short to work in a place of misery and deal with sickness at the same time.

Phew... in making this decision I felt an enormous weight lift from my shoulders and years of stress were released from within me. It was as if another person had been literally standing on top of me these past nine months (with no shoes on, of course, I would say probably bare smelly feet).

Jude and I decided to take a well-earned holiday that we came across in one of those deals you get bombarded with by email, and so we planned to fly to Fiji for an eight-day vacation. Our online travel deal included a four-star hotel, breakfast, wines and dinner. It would give us the opportunity to clear our heads and forget about everything going on in Sydney for the time being. I also had the thumbs up from Dr. Susan as long as I didn't go scuba diving and deep-water swimming so as to avoid the sharp coral.

A trip to Fiji was just what we needed at this time. The weather was hot, but not humid and the locals were hospitable and friendly with the food being excellent. My experience with workplace bullying faded to the back of my mind, along with my low blood platelet count. But seven days goes very quickly and after an amazing week away I went straight into treatment upon my return.

More tests were carried out by the hospital when I arrived back into Sydney. This regime of testing seemingly went on for weeks and weeks, including a very painful biopsy, which was taken from just below my belly button.

Career

My career as a chef first began after I completed a two-year full-time course in catering. This career path developed while working at five-star hotels in London such as The Grosvenor House and the Hilton Hotel on Park Lane, which were followed by a stint in a Casino and a few restaurants.

Not long after my arrival in Sydney, I worked at the Sydney Convention Centre and the corporate section of Sydney Football Stadium at Moore Park. I alternated between these two positions for a full ten years. After this, I moved on to working in catering companies, the aged care industry and for a private hospital.

My background was in catering and I had trained and worked

hard to become a catering chef, which I became quite experienced in over the past 15 years. The establishment I was posted at were in need of a kitchen manager, so as I was already helping out there, I applied for and was lucky enough to win the job. To be honest, initially it was an industry I knew precious little about, apart from six months I once spent working in an aged care establishment, which wasn't at all easy.

Watching the residents in aged care, I often reflected on how humans arrive in this world requiring much love, nurturing and direction with some occasional assistance from nappies. Then towards the end of our life, most of us also require much love, nurturing and direction with some occasional assistance from nappies!!!

At this establishment, my duties were to prepare a selection of tasty, but not spicy soft textured easily palatable foods. I also had to prepare specific diets for patients with swallowing difficulties and special diets, and supervising other less qualified staff was a component of the position.

It was at work that my problems began when I gradually became aware of frequent work issues developing between myself and my immediate supervisor, which occurred over an extended period. I believe in hard work and I put a lot of effort into what I do, but there should be fair and equitable procedures for dealing with issues and conflicts that arise from time to time. However, I very early on found myself to be the target of workplace bullying, which I later learnt was unfortunately quite common in this industry.

A continuous barrage of meetings between the supervisor, mediators and myself didn't do anything to resolve the issues and it began to affect me on a deeper level. I began experiencing a lack of sleep due to stress and worry and then rapidly began to lose weight. Even though I ate the same amount daily and trained at the gym, my weight started to plummet.

The problem was that each working day was like walking on eggshells, I found it difficult to relax and my mind started playing tricks with me. I would second guess everything I did, even simple tasks I had performed hundreds of times. For example, when braising meat for a stew, or simply frying fish, my mind would be subjected to a virtual game of tennis... "do it like this Joseph! No! do it like that Joseph. Your boss won't like it, your boss will like it..." it was painstakingly exhausting, I felt constantly fatigued and even fearful, especially on my way to work.

Each morning my stomach churned itself into a large knot, causing butterflies and anxiety at the prospect of facing another day as a work victim. There is only so much bullying one can take before it begins to show its effect. I can recall when my boss tried to turn the kitchen staff against me by putting words in their mouths within the safe confines of her office. There were never any witnesses but always a high level of intimidation. I knew this because the staff members who had been questioned by this supervisor told me first hand about this attempted intimidation.

No matter what time I went to bed I would toss and turn, thinking about the day's events and what problems I'd have to face tomorrow. Having hardly slept I would wake up exhausted on a daily basis. Acne was first introduced into my world at 14 years old and now decided to pay me another visit in my thirties. Luckily they showed themselves as single 'zits', not in a cluster like a bunch of berries.

I only wanted to be heard at work and felt the way I had been treated was both unprofessional and unfair. So I decided to go over my supervisors head and share my difficult situation directly with human resources, who often intervened. Not surprisingly, for a few weeks following each intervention my boss left me quite alone and even acknowledged me when we came across each other in the corridor. But I didn't trust her at all and tried to avoid her altogether if possible.

I recalled a dé-jà-vu moment from back when I was a pupil in junior school, doing what any guilty pupil would do to avoid a super strict Principal. Whether they were a Mr., Mrs., Miss or Ms. they typically had a fake smile, zero tolerance and would always give out detentions for something we thought was absolutely trivial.

This kind of negative thinking was very repetitive and played on my mind every time I ran into my boss. The food for the kitchen had to be ordered through a computer and special phone system, which was located only 20 metres from her office. I came to despise this particular task because of the proximity it drew both of us into.

CHAPTER 2

The Struggle Ahead

Round One

Dr. Susan was the head of the department and seemed to be solely in charge of my case. As time went on we got to know each other very well. She often joked and once commented that I was the talk of the specialist team of doctors in meetings at the hospital. The apparent reason was that there was a mystery concerning my low platelets, and what caused them in the first place. My particular symptoms didn't line up within any probable diagnosis. Then I received a memorable, but dreaded phone call from Dr. Susan.

"Joseph can you please come into my office at the hospital when you can, we have the results from your biopsy. Are you available tomorrow at noon?" She asked.

We all know that whenever it is bad news the doctor rings and says... "I would like you to come into my office". This drama is played out frequently in the movies, TV dramas and reality TV shows, but now it was actually happening to me. My mind started racing, asking a never ending list of questions. The workplace bullying saga came back to me and I heard the sound of drums. Although I couldn't see the drummer, my heart was beating so hard I could definitely hear him. That night was a restless one indeed.

Next day my wife Jude went with me to the appointment for support, to share the load (as she put it) that was about to be dropped on my head like a ton of bricks. As soon as we walked into my haematologist's office (I say 'my haematologist' because Dr. Susan and I were now going to be seeing a lot of each other), Dr. Susan instructed me to sit and she looked worriedly into my eyes. After four months of tests, all the questions and appointments had come to an abrupt end as I braced myself for what the doctor had to say.

"Joseph, your biopsy results show that you have enlarged lymph nodes of three to five centimetres in diameter around your groin and stomach area. We have reason to believe that you have contracted a rare case of Hodgkin's Lymphoma".

I had heard that name before, but didn't know what it meant. She went on to say... "It will be necessary for you to receive six to eight sessions of radiation to eradicate them".

Bang... well, you could have shot me with a canon. Now I was really worried! I felt numb and couldn't move. My mind became overactive thinking of what this all meant. Radiation meant cancer didn't it? Oh no, Oh No... questions raced around my head like a formula one Grand Prix final.

For the next 30 minutes or so I honestly cannot remember what else we talked about, it all became just a blur. Dr. Susan was perfectly calm and professional as she spoke, and had obviously delivered this talk to many other patients over the years. I tried to remain calm, but I was scared. I glanced over at Jude and noticed her facial expression had become one of fear and panic.

I eventually blurted out...

"About the radiation, do I have any other choices?" The answer was both clear and very blunt...

"You can leave it, but you won't get any better, in fact the lymph nodes will get even bigger if you do nothing about them!"

It was all a huge shock and very hard to realise that I, of all people, had contracted cancer. But, after I calmed down a little I was somewhat reassured by Dr. Susan that there would be minimal side effects from the regime of treatments. She also mentioned that there was often a good success rate and few complications.

The radiation sessions started the first week of January 2011 and were carried out for 30 minutes each time. After five sessions I became very sick and extremely nauseated, which in turn led me to refusing treatment, and I admit becoming a very difficult patient with the oncology team. I would start to vomit as soon as I entered the hospital, and demanded to speak to the head of oncology because I didn't want any more treatment. They reluctantly agreed to this request and placed me on temporary hold.

But as it turned out the halt in the treatment just delayed the inevitable, as the halt in the daily treatments just delayed the entire cycle. Hence two months became three months and it was as though I had been possessed by a demon. However, throughout the treatments the oncology staff remained very understanding and patient. When it was finally over I apologized to them for my stubbornness and difficult behaviour.

The side effects I suffered were a loss of appetite and I suffered from emotional nausea. But most noticeable was a severe loss of weight as I lost seven kilograms within a very short time. All in all, it took my body six months to overcome the accumulated side effects of the procedures I experienced and the medication I had to consume. Luckily, the lymph nodes were greatly reduced in size and stopped growing. But, I mistakenly thought that was the end of it, which sadly was not to be the case.

At this time in my life I was working as a chef at three separate catering venues, all on a consistently casual basis. I would work for whichever venue offered me the most hours that week or month. The work in Sydney was plentiful especially when I first arrived from

England. Chefs were hard to procure so quite most of us would pick and choose our days and organise work hours to suit. I found that by committing to one venue, you could easily fit in the other two and regularly work five days a week on casual wages. In fact, on many of these days there were even double shifts available.

Round Two

How I developed cancer for a second time, and how suffering crept back into my life was both insidious and terrifying.

I had to repair damage to a torn rotator cuff in my left shoulder, which occurred at work. At this time I was working as a catering delivery driver and was required to carry heavy loads of food and alcohol on a regular basis. The wear and tear on my shoulder resulted in the rotator cuff injury.

Four weeks after the surgery I started experiencing an agonizing shooting pain from my buttocks all the way down my legs. I only felt the pain when I laid down, and it became so bad that I couldn't lie down at all or sit still for more than three hours without the pain becoming excruciating. I asked myself "Was this where the saying came from... 'It's a pain in the butt'?" My only relief from the suffering came when standing or walking around. This episode lasted for ten long days and even longer nights with sleep being virtually non-existent, so naturally my temper became very short.

The thoughts in my head played continuously like a CD, from start to finish. In the beginning I murmured to myself... "Joseph you are an African Zulu warrior who feels no pain and fights to the bitter end". Then when I could no longer stand it, I'd ask myself "what are you doing going round and round in circles"? I tried to mentally block out the pain and just lie down, put my feet up and convince myself that this was all in my mind. However, I had to cave in to the pain and I whimpered like a young puppy whose owner has gone to work for the day and whilst you're at it, it wee'd all over the new carpet.

My local general practitioner suggested a series of cortisone injections below my spine because oral painkillers may not have any effect. He also issued me with a referral letter, which introduced me to a radiologist using my 'medicare card'. This meant I could qualify for a rebate from the government. Without the rebate the consultation would have cost quite a lot, as I had just used up all my work entitlements to recover from the shoulder operation.

Booking through a hospital required a three month waiting list, but medicare shortened the wait and it was a great relief for me to look forward to a possible solution at last. With Cortisone injections everyone has a different response. Approximately one third of patients get no relief, one-third get some temporary relief and the final third have a fantastic reaction, where the pain doesn't return.

I had to undergo a series of three injections, over five days. The radiologist admitted it was a challenge to hit the exact spot because my back and spine area were continuously in spasm as the needle entered my skin. Anyway it worked straight away, which was a great victory for now.

Sometimes God sends angels and helpers down to earth to guide and help us. After listening to my non sleep dilemma I felt this doctor was sent to help me. His name was Dr. Moses and he instructed the receptionist to charge me a reduced fee, which in my mind was icing on the cake on both counts. I could now sleep, lie down, relax and I felt so relieved to be able to live a normal life, which is otherwise generally taken for granted.

But, what disturbed me most was a burning issue in my mind. What actually caused this episode to happen in the first place? I was suspicious that something so painful could just suddenly occur, so were there any lingering issues from my earlier battle with cancer?

I had to undergo more tests, scans involving a PET scan, which stands for Positron Emission Tomography. This method uses radiation or nuclear medicine imaging to provide unique information about how an organ or system in the body is working. This is one of the most effective ways to view any ongoing problems with soft tissue. My local hospital had none of these machines so I was referred to the Royal Prince Alfred Hospital in Sydney. The results took a week to process, which meant another visit to Dr. Susan for the results.

After consulting my personal advisor, 'Dr. Google on Wikipedia', I was totally convinced that my problem could be sorted out with some acupuncture or a number of visits to a chiropractor. Of course my haematologist told me differently. I wasn't prepared in any way shape or form for what Dr. Susan was about to tell me.

She began..."Joseph you have a very rare and aggressive type of Hodgkins Lymphoma, which has returned. There were only four types of your particular strain that were detected amongst literally hundreds tested over last years' studies."

She went on to say... "You have a Nodular Lymphocyte Predominant type, slower growing than the classical Hodgkins Lymphoma". I thought to myself... "I hope the cancer knows that?" Dr. Susan continued... "If not treated could grow bigger and more aggressive, at which stage you may not be able to treat it at all."

I was absolutely gutted with a capital G!! "No, No, NOOO, Not Again!" Was I supposed to be comforted by the fact that I was now a unique person, with a unique condition, facing a unique death... Hmmmm??

My mind went haywire, thoughts splattered all over my head, the same way a sand blaster is used on a construction site! To give you an idea, my mouth was wide open like a goldfish gulping, but I couldn't form any words. Sweat started to gather in all my gland areas, my doctor's words faded in then out like waves washing up on a beach.

After what seemed like a lifetime, my pent up reaction finally blurted out of me... "Didn't the six weeks of daily radiation last year kill it? You know, the one where the side-effects made me sick for months afterwards?"

"No" my Doctor replied, "although the radiation slowed it down, it is an aggressive type and over the course of the past 12 to 18 months it has obviously started to grow again. You will need chemotherapy to kill it this time around." I could feel myself becoming aggressive.

"But can't I just have another course of radiation?" I belted out. I couldn't believe that came out of my mouth especially after what I'd previously been through! We wrestled back and forth for a compromise, with my Doctor offering solutions and suggestions, whilst I opposed everything she threw at me. Finally we sort of came to a truce with which I was given a few days to go home, think about it and come back to her with a decision.

She suggested that I undertake anywhere from six to eight chemotherapy treatments, depending on the consulting oncologist (cancer specialist). Each individual chemotherapy session would be undertaken every second Monday, depending if I felt well enough to continue, with a normal chemotherapy session usually lasting between five and six hours. What could I do? After mulling it over, I didn't really have a choice as it was obviously serious, so I had to agree to the treatment.

The date was December 2012, and the oncology team wanted to get started almost straight away. I stood in front of an abyss of fear, the unknown was staring me in the face. For all those original Star Trek fans 'I was going where no Joseph Anaman had ever gone before' and I was very, very scared. Not about the disease, but I was about to enter a place I knew very little about.

I frantically searched the internet, chat forums and articles on how people normally reacted to treatment after contracting this kind of disease. But, I couldn't find anything... Nada! I felt depleted, exhausted and quite angry that a full description of a chemotherapy cycle and how a person feels and reacts throughout such a treatment was not available. But what was I really looking for anyway as last time around, the radiation felt terrible most of the time!

"Overall I don't know what all the fuss was about"... I told myself "it would be a breeze!" But perhaps, I was just trying to fool myself. I eventually came across some real data and concluded that everyone suffers the side effects of chemotherapy in different ways. Most felt sick at some point, some lost weight and a few even put on weight. But no matter what their genetic make up, virtually everyone suffered, they just responded differently.

Two days later I agreed to go through with the recommended treatment, knowing that I wouldn't be alone on this journey. My wife Jude, my family, my friends and acquaintances and most importantly, my God would be walking with me. Now that I'd decided to follow the recommended course of action, when would all my troubles go away?

CHAPTER 3

Fighting Back

Tests

The first test procedure I needed to undergo was to have a heart assessment, which under normal conditions takes around 45 minutes. When I was informed about this test, I decided to put myself through a grueling four week fitness and cross-training regime. As it turned out, what a waste of time that was. I was thinking I'd sit for the test by pedaling on a stationary bike, with loads of wires attached to various body parts, I'd be sweating, huffing and puffing. I thought alongside me would be a doctor in their white lab coat, instructing me to eat less carbs, watch my diet and stop smoking.

But the heart fitness test was quite the opposite. It consisted merely of a resting heart monitor, a few photographs, a blood test and the insertion of fluid into my system. I actually fell asleep during the test. It was just too much excitement for one day... NOT! However, at least I had built up my level of fitness for what lay ahead.

The next test protocol was much more invasive. It was a bone marrow biopsy. I was given some laughing gas through a type of whistle and asked to slowly breathe through it, to ease the pain. When I was deemed to be in a sufficiently numb state, a large needle was jabbed vertically into my hip, which I felt hit the bone, it was then twisted and a piece of bone marrow was extracted.

As painful as it sounds, this procedure wasn't too bad, just a bit uncomfortable on the nerves. The medical assistant who was doing the extracting was breaking sweat, as he heaved at my hip for maybe ten minutes or so.

End Of The Beginning

TREATMENT 1

Before reaching the age of 40, I would have been able to count on one hand how many times I'd been inside a hospital. I hadn't ever suffered broken bones, concussions or mysterious diseases forcing me to get up in the middle of the night, to spend a few hours sitting in cold emergency departments.

Then five years ago I felt something inside me start to change, when the joints in my hips started to lock up and I felt the first signs of what I thought were wear and tear from aging. But, that was not the case. What happened next descended upon me so rapidly, it made my head spin.

It all began with three months of consultations with oncology specialists trying to figure out what kind of growth was developing in my lower abdomen. Then... Bang! My rotator cuffs muscles in both shoulders started to ache after suffering tears of some seven to eleven centimeters long. Bang again! The growth in my abdomen duplicated itself in a different location, causing me weeks of excruciating pain and broken sleep almost every night. Going back into hospital wasn't easy, but I faced it with strength and resolve. I was determined not to allow this experience to take a hold over me. I tried to pump myself up by remembering the lyrics to a simple song, while walking down the corridors of the hospital. Pharell Williams had composed a song called "Happy," which was a wonderful feel-good song. If you ever happened to catch the video clip, not only would your feet start tapping, but your whole face would be smiling.

Humming this song to myself I passed by a young guy in his twenties walking on crutches, who was in distress with a bandaged foot, a young child coughing continuously in the arms of her mother, and a workman holding a bandaged and bloodied hand. Hospitals were never the most uplifting places to spend time.

As I got into the elevator, my heart started pumping twice as loud, as if it was going to jump right out of my chest. My pulse quickened, perspiration appeared on my brow. Out of the elevator a small girl around the age of seven was being pushed in a wheelchair, her face was one of pure innocence, but her slumped body looked frail and her skin was a pale, lifeless colour.

So why was I here, again, inexplicably about to start yet another journey? I quite naturally became increasingly concerned about the personal journey that lay ahead. Through chance meetings with similarly affected people, I had the presence of mind and the strong urge to want to record my personal battle with Hodgkin's Lymphoma. So, not knowing whether I could maintain it, or whether I would even be around to keep it going, I resolved to keep a diary of my daily experiences. The journey and my reflections were recorded as often as I could handle under the circumstances.

The first day of treatment was a milestone in the journey as it marked the point at which the doubts and mental anguish of having developed HL, gave way to a means by which this life-threatening disease could possibly be cured. It was in my eyes, the end of the beginning!

The chemotherapy process went like this. First up, my blood pulse and temperature were taken followed by the recording of my weight and height statistics. A tube is then fed through a bottle hanging upside down, which is attached to a stand and a solution known as R-Chop is fed through an intravenous drip into my system through a cannula or IV, which passes into my veins located on either hand.

Then follows Rituximab (an antibody) as a slow infusion. In fact, I can recall that my very first infusion of Rituximab took around four and a half hours. The catheter was placed into my vein with great care and the pace of the infusion was always very slow. After that Cyclophosphamide is given as a fast infusion, and finally Vinicristine as a push dose into the drip also as a slow infusion.

Prednisone tablets are taken for the first five days after every cycle. On the second day following my cycle I inject myself through the folds of my stomach with Neulasta. The nursing staff showed me how to administer this treatment. I also take home Ondansetron wafers to help with nausea and Nexium to help with stomach reflux.

This was the medication process I had to undergo for each cycle or treatment. The first time I was issued with Prednisone was in 2010 for up to four months when my blood platelets were low. After this was my radiotherapy for a few months.

At the end of each chemotherapy session I slept for what seemed like hours, the duration of treatment being for four hours. I guess digesting those chemicals into my system and killing off the unwanted growths took its toll on my body.

The very first treatment consisted of me being exposed to a medical procedure that was identified by the abbreviation of 'R-Chop.' Upon hearing this frightful term I thought to myself "what an unwelcoming and inappropriate name for such a life threatening procedure." It was kind of like having to undergo 'rhinoplasty' (another incredulous term) for a nose job, and I wondered if rhino's had been the original patients?

Nursing staff always closely observed the patients, especially the first-timers. I felt a bit like a 'VIP', a very important patient! Routine checks and blood pressure were taken regularly. Then, the next three infusions were given. All together, a marathon nine hours passed by.

The next day, although tired and with a stomach upset in the morning, I otherwise felt fine. Jude and I went to see a french movie called "The Intouchables," which was witty, humorous and very entertaining. The story reflected two men from completely different backgrounds filling each other's voids. We laughed throughout and really enjoyed the flick.

It was Friday, the end of my first week and I felt OK at first, but as the day progressed I started to become a bit 'dodgy' here and there. This went on all day and through into the night. I found out early on that nausea mixed with a hot, humid day was not a good combination for my condition at all! The next two to three days were very, very uncomfortable. I felt queasy, nauseous and constantly had an upset stomach.

Four days into the treatment I suddenly perked up. Day four was the best I had felt all week. I woke up as usual with the alarm, but decided to get back into bed for those precious five minutes we all like to have on workdays.

I felt surprisingly good on my first day back at work since my treatment began, despite knowing that the chemotherapy treatments were to span another three months.

My haematologist had warned me that as the treatment wore on my body would also become more worn down. As I hadn't experienced this aggressive and deadly form of disease before, the logical thing was to take each day or week as it came, and just try to tough it out. But not knowing what was around the corner made me feel both helpless and vulnerable.

As a family my thoughts turned to how would we survive through this ordeal? I knew we had bills and expenses to fork out like everyone else, but we didn't want to get ourselves in debt, our credit cards had already reached their limit. We did have money saved for a rainy day, but it was not a great amount by any means. I wasn't a teenager who would be able to turn to his parents for advice or financial support when the going got tough, nor was I a pensioner whose family would come to the rescue. I was bang in the middle, with a wife and daughter to support. These financial worries added to my health burden, which meant that giving up work was entirely out of the question.

We were situated in that class just above poverty, but well below middle class, living from week to week, from pay cheque to pay cheque. I've never been one to shy away from work, and I couldn't leave the financial pressure solely with my wife Jude. I had a role to play in my marriage, I had always been the breadwinner, plus my profession paid a little more due to my accumulated experience.

A Blessing

Jude and I had always been spiritual people and have been members at our local church for about ten years now. Since then and even before, our hearts had always been willing to help others who were doing it tough or going through difficult times. During those ten years we had built up great relationships and had accumulated some really good friends.

The culture our church adopted too, was one to rally round and pull together in unity. When our church friends found out about my cancer and treatment, Lee and Craige took it upon themselves to go to the church members. They suggested that for anyone who was willing and able to help, to contribute a love financial offering to assist us through our troubles. This extremely kind gesture was to help my family and myself through this situation without worrying about finances, and especially for when I felt too ill to work. The timing couldn't have been better, at this stage I was halfway through my first treatment and each day started as a surprise package. I never quite knew what the next hour would bring.

This was for us an unbelievable gesture of love. We were so grateful to everyone and personally thanked each individual who contributed and were a part of this wonderful gift. We have so many memories and blessings during our lifetime as well as trials and struggles, but when I am in a good space, which is most of the time, the fondest memories are never forgotten and gestures such as this were definitely one of them.

> *Remember this: Whoever sows sparingly will reap sparingly, and whoever sows generously will also reap generously. Each man should give what he has decided in his heart to give, not reluctantly or under compulsion, for God loves a cheerful giver. And God is able to make all grace abound to you, so that in all things, at all times, having all that you need, you will abound in every good work. As it is written: He has scattered abroad his gifts to the poor; his righteousness endures forever.*
>
> *2 Corinthians 9:6-10*

On my way to work, I usually turned the car radio on and did my compulsory channel surfing between the different FM stations, before eventually settling on a catchy song. Still very tired, but otherwise feeling good I'd find myself singing along, quite loudly I may add to songs like "Slow Down" by Bobby Valentino.

I didn't usually start my day at 5:30am in this manner, but for some strange reason I often felt really good in the mornings. Next, I'd belted out the chorus (with changed words) of an Eminem song. "Guess who's back, back again. Joseph's back, tell your friends."

The next few days felt like a mixture of an experience at being one of the winning contestants walking through a room at Willy Wonka's Chocolate Factory, then being immediately catapulted into a Dungeon of Doom, before taking a trip to Wet n' Wild. Let me try to explain.

As each child experienced a room at Willy Wonka's Chocolate Factory their level of intensity would fluctuate from surprise to bewilderment, in awe of the delicious, edible lollies, which could be consumed by simply falling to the ground and chewing the countryside. This is how I often felt in the morning... excited and full of beans.

Then there would be a down turn when the nausea and stomach acid hit me. I would be consumed by an ordeal of distress and torment. Emotion bore down on me, and I would become sorrowful and helpless. I could compare the feeling of the chemo spreading itself throughout my system to a 'Wet n' Wild' adventure ride with profuse sweating and heat suffocating my entire body just like being a hot and humid, tropical Queensland climate. After which, my powerful thirst would be quenched with copious amounts of water.

It was around this time that I developed a serious case of indigestion, which gave me a very unpleasant nights sleep, interrupted by a few midnight trips to the toilet. The reason for this was that one of my medication packs caused fluid retention in the body. After the last meal of an evening, I normally felt a little peckish, but not on these nights. This particular medication created a stomach upset, and I could feel mouth ulcers starting to develop. I thought to myself "here we go!"

These feelings of being physically uncomfortable gradually developed into an easily recognizable routine. It would start with nausea first thing in the morning, which left me with absolutely no appetite. I felt sluggish and didn't want to converse with anyone. Then within an hour I would turn into a chatterbox and chew anyone's ear off. Shortly after that, paranoia would get a grip on me, resulting in me crawling back into a uncommunicative shell.

An hour later, nausea would pay another visit, the remedy for which was simply small snacks. Snacking seemed to stop my stomach acid from entering the back of my throat by providing the acid with something to consume other than me! Whenever the stomach acid became too much, vomiting would start and I'd experience bouts of profuse sweating and feelings of being hot and humid.

I'd wonder if the air temperature was getting too hot or was it just me. So I'd often take a look at the people around me like my wife Jude, my daughter or my work colleagues' foreheads and faces. "What, no sweating?" I'd asked my mates, "do any of you feel hot?" when the temperature was really quite mild. Then I'd develop a craving thirst, so much so that when I finally arrived home from work at around 4pm, I'd spend the next two hours downing literally liters of fluids to quench my thirst.

This nauseating sequence of nasty effects would repeat themselves again in the early afternoon. When sitting quietly of an evening I often felt strong pain in my left hip, which came from where I'd previously had the bone marrow removed. It was no comfort that my specialist did warn me that this could happen, but the only solution to relieve the discomfort was to take a painkiller. I always did my best to ignore my hip discomfort, hoping it would go away and it eventually did.

I felt so good on one particular day that I even went to the gym. The desire was definitely there, but my intensity and energy levels quickly dropped off, which I discovered about 15 minutes into my workout. After the workout I was so spent that I even took a quick dip in the swimming pool, an unusual event for me.

Do you know what was so odd about that? Well, our swimming pool at home is located just two meters from the back door. The pool had been ready and cleaned regularly by our good friends Joseph and Paula for the past two months. I normally just glanced at it, thinking to myself... "Ooh that looks refreshing", but I'd normally walk past it, and then go upstairs. But, not on this particular day, when I felt like Superman. I plunged in, with Eminem playing again in my head, "Joseph is back, back again."

I had felt a bit heady one particular day, meaning I felt foggy-minded, my judgment was cloudy and I wasn't quite present in the company of others. I thought to myself that if I were a practicing psychologist or counsellor today, I'd have to reverse roles with my clients, or give them their money back. It would be me sitting in the warm, comfy, leather chair receiving some kind of therapy and not the other way round!

These were just some of the side-effects that became obvious to me on a day to day basis. To help me overcome the constant problems, I got into the habit of murmuring the following prayer:

Oh Lord do not forsake me
Be not far from me Oh my Lord
Come quickly to help me
Oh Lord my saviour

Psalm 38: 21-22

CHAPTER 4

The Grind

Sustenance

Every day is a challenge of some sort in everyone's life, whether it's mild or severe, positive or negative, but the challenges I faced changed from day to day. I recall one particular day when the challenge that confronted me was body odour, but thankfully not my own! I had been noticing all kinds of changes were happening to me since I started treatment, but began noticing that my nasal senses were becoming increasingly acute.

On one day, I was asked to supervise and work alongside a casual employee in the kitchen, who had a bad, no, very bad, case of body odour! It turned out to be a very challenging morning. When I say we worked 'alongside,' that's exactly how it was. As a chef, this person had to be physically next to me, to observe every task I performed. The debilitating experience lasted six whole hours. It would be fair of me to say that on that day I expressed at least 100 different ways of pulling a face without physically vomiting.

On the flip side, I really began to enjoy fresh fruit and found that nectarines, lychees, mangoes and strawberries smelt divine, were really refreshing and tasted better than ever.

On another morning we all had to begin work an hour earlier, and a 5am start isn't easy at the very best of times. My left eye was bloodshot, and I felt a bit heady, but in patches throughout the day. When my co-workers asked me what was wrong I commented on the early start and asked them never to roster me on at such an unearthly time. I was half joking, but sometimes jokes have an underlying truth.

That afternoon I had intentions of attending my friend's annual Christmas party. Thirty minutes prior to leaving for the party, I shut my eyes and woke up two hours later. Needless to say, I didn't go. It would have been fun socially and great to catch up with my friend, but my body told me to rest and mentally I really wasn't up to it.

The weekend arrived and I felt like I was back to my usual self. I puttered around the house and sang to myself an old Jimmy Cliff song, but slightly altered the lyrics:

> "I can see clearly now the fog has gone!
> I can see all obstacles in my way.
> Gone is the nausea that had me down
> It's gonna be a bright, bright, bright sunshinin' day!"

Problem was, I just didn't have the normal stamina, and I couldn't help noticing how my energy levels would quickly deteriorate throughout a day. I felt like one of those toy dolls when their batteries were completely depleted and they ran out of power! But the one thing I could do very well was rest and I made sure I recharged whenever I could.

Routine

Unfortunately, Mondays always came around way too fast and the working week would start again. But I knew the bills weren't going to stop and that thought was enough to get me to roll out of bed and gather the energy to begin my normal daily routine. As the day wore on, I felt whatever energy I had brought to work, would quickly deteriorate throughout the day.

Lunch couldn't ever come quick enough. Even though I spend most of my day in a commercial kitchen, a lunchbox always accompanied me at work. It was a habit that had stuck with me for years. Just like a young toddler who carries their favorite toy or blanket with them around their home. My work colleagues will tell you that I won't ever turn up for work without my little blue lunchbox in hand. Why blue? Because a pink one would of course clash with my chefs uniform.

Inside my lunchbox I usually carried an assortment of snacks, fresh fruit, possibly a poached chicken sandwich, or takeaway containers with pasta or rice mixed with canned tuna. I always tried to keep my lunch simple, but in sufficient quantities. Why? Well, you might know the saying, "Never trust a skinny chef!"

The real reason I carried so much food with me was that I had a very fast metabolism, which required me to snack every three to four hours. I honestly think that if I resorted to three large meals a day, which isn't advised by dietitians anyway, that I'd collapse in a heap with stomach cramp or hunger pain.

Even though my diet was simple, I was a fussy bugger when it came to food variety and choices. Unless I cooked it myself, I didn't ever order a steak from any other food place. The disappointments I've suffered over the years were just too many to mention. Unless I cooked them myself the only pancakes I ever ordered were from 'Pancakes On The Rocks', and beef ribs only ever came from the bar and grill called 'Hurricanes.'

When I see or hear about food critics, a part of me says "I'd love that job." Then the other part of me, which is my real self coming through says "No you wouldn't!" You see, not every meal is a winner. Some dishes can absolutely blow my socks off, but others will leave you feeling terribly disappointed. So I wouldn't want to go home with my head down and my tail between my legs, knowing that critics out there frequently report on how chefs regularly botch up perfectly good ingredients.

My loss of energy continued, so much so that directly after lunch I found myself struggling to do anything constructive at all. I would often reach inside my lunchbox and pull out a bottle of Powerade to see if that could invigorate me. Within 60 minutes of consuming my drink however, I always felt somewhat better and this carried me through most afternoons.

Upon reaching home, instead of my power nap being the usual 15-20 minutes, it would stretch out to 90-120 minutes and I'd awake in a sleepy stupor. I knew this behaviour was very unusual for me and these were obviously the side-effects kicking in.

Nausea

One of my medications had reduced from 100 mg a day, over the past few months to gradually zero. This particular medication was called Prednisone, which acted as an inflammatory to boost my red blood cells. By this time I had been on Prednisone for the past four months. The Prednisone tablets were taken daily, the effects of which were not so apparent for me to notice, except that it stimulated my appetite, causing me to feel ravenous most of the day, which in turn caused me to quickly put on weight. At times I even asked myself "was I pregnant and didn't know it?"

For those who have never watched the movie 'The Nutty Professor', let me describe how I went through my own transformation and changed characters from a 'Buddy Love' type into a kind of 'Professor Clump', in a real and very physical way.

I make this comparison because it is interesting, that at this point quite a few people I met commented on how much I looked like Eddie Murphy. Even on our most recent family holiday, where I got a strange look from one of the immigration officers as I joined the arriving passengers customs line.

We all know it's their job to screen everyone and give people a cold hard stare. But, I reckon it's all tactics so we passengers start to perspire, shake and fumble around for our passports in front of them. Then they ask...

"Why are you acting so suspiciously? What are you guilty of? or, Are you hiding something?"

Of course if we don't give the right answers we get whisked off to a detaining room and have our bags searched, and possibly even strip-searched. I think they'd absolutely have to love their job! I'm sure that morning tea in their staff room would be a daily laugh in, discussing what is found in various peoples' luggage being the source of much entertainment over their cup of coffee.

Anyway, this Immigration Officer and I got talking, but she had to double-check my passport before telling me she honestly believed I was Eddie Murphy, and she was even going to ask me for an autograph. We all laughed and my wife thought it so amusing that she shared it with anyone she spoke to for the entire month. This coincidence to the famous Hollywood star happens often, but that's another story.

Back to how I turned into 'Professor Clump' from taking Prednisone. This medication caused a number of side-effects including: fluid retention and bloating in my face and stomach particularly; constant emptying of the bladder and broken sleep; anxiety, making it hard for me to settle into any sleep pattern; spots on my shoulders and face; frequent indigestion causing me great discomfort; increased appetite, which resulted in me spending too much time in the kitchen preparing food and eating; a big, bulging stomach; and to top it off I had heartburn every day, which became worse in the middle of the night.

This medication had to be taken at the beginning of each chemotherapy cycle. Whoopee! But despite living with these afflicting side-effects, I felt relatively OK on the majority of days.

But, I pondered that if each cycle was going to be like this, I couldn't see how I was ever going to cope. Little did I know, that this was just the start of my journey and that I was in for the ride of my life!

For I am the Lord, your God, who takes hold of your right hand and says to you, Do not fear; for I will help you.

Isiah 41: 13-14

I could tolerate pain to a certain degree, but nausea was a completely different story. I've tried, but me and nausea just don't get along at all. There is absolutely no compromise! The instant I felt it, even the way the word sounded, I lost my appetite and my patience. When I was experiencing nausea, it caused a knock-on effect right throughout my body, but it particularly affected my sense of:

- Taste, as food has no taste and becomes undesirable.
- Smell, with every aroma and scent is heightened tenfold.
- Sight, which creates a feeling of vulnerability.
- Touch, causing uncertainty and a loss of confidence.
- Hearing, with sound often muffled causing a confusion.

Needless to say, our senses are relied upon on a daily basis and although most of us take them for granted, unbeknown to me, my sense organs were about to take an absolute battering.

The hospital was a boring place at the best of times. Apart from daytime television, my only other source of entertainment was watching the goings on in the hospital itself. What else could I do for up to nine hours at a time?

One morning whilst waiting for my particular treatment, I sat next to a fellow patient. He looked like he had experienced a hard time with his health, the chemo or perhaps both. His eyes were vacant, he was gaunt looking, possibly in his 50's, short hair in patches, which was probably due to the multiple treatments he'd undergone. I overheard his blood pressure reading was 90 over 50.

I got the feeling that this very low reading was part of a regular cycle for him over the last two to three years. On this day however, he refused treatment, stating he was just too sick following his last visit. His previous consultation had been a month prior and the chemo cycle was apparently far too aggressive for his body, which he determinedly asserted needed a rest. The nurses went back and forth seeking their supervisor and then talked with him. It reminded me of a game of tennis that went on for what seemed like a whole tennis match. Eventually they sent the patient home.

CHAPTER 5

Keeping Sane

The Weed

During my frequent visits to the hospital I met a fellow patient who had already experienced a few years of chemotherapy. I didn't know his name, but he was a teacher who had previously worked in Japan and Vietnam. He recalled that his tumour had initially appeared below his left ear, but apart from small patches of hair loss and the uneven colour of his skin, he otherwise looked fine.

However, six months later, like most of these pesky buggers, his tumour made an unwelcome return. To battle the new growth his next dose of 'chemo' was much stronger, because his tumour had been diagnosed as being much more aggressive. His personal side-effects were vomiting and bouts of fitting, but up to that point he was completely unaware that he was pre-disposed to epilepsy.

A few years later, after many treatments, he returned to Sydney and this was when we met, but he hadn't been able to work over the previous few months. He told me that after just three treatments into his chemotherapy, vomiting was usually brought induced, but only on the first day. However, right from the start, fatigue and tiredness restricted him to being a virtual prisoner in his own home.

Feeling familiar with each other, it was at this point that he decided to broach the subject. He asked... "Do you ever smoke the weed?' To which I instinctually answered... "No!" Although I knew that wasn't really the case. He then went on to explain in detail how 'the weed' had helped him on his low days. I quickly thanked him for sharing his chemo experience with me as he was being called into the treatment room. After a few hours had passed, he emerged and on leaving he bade me good-bye and whispered, "Remember the weed!"

My initial introduction to the magical properties of marijuana was in Australia through a family acquaintance named John, who grew his own and reaped the rewards. In fact, the weed and myself go back a long way. You could say we were mates, buddies, business partners. We even shared a house together!

He had a government job and supported his family as best he could. However, he reasoned that without getting too greedy, making a little 'pocket money' on the side could relieve the day-to-day pressures of an average working family, helping them cope and put a bounce in their step. Obviously, it can all turn pear-shaped if people become too greedy. His goal and heart's desire was to buy his own home and live off the land with just his family and livestock to care for.

He shared some interesting tips and assured me that his mother plant was in a very well-manicured state. To me it was like comparing the cultivation of a prized plant with the development of a champion thoroughbred racehorse. I am sure top breeders believe that their best horses bear champions.

He once shared with me a maths equation or formula, depending on which way you chose to define it, of how much can be made from one ounce to one pound of 'weed'. The business strategy depended solely upon the number of people involved.

With a one man operation you could have plenty of customers and returns can be quick and plentiful. However you may also develop plenty of enemies. With more business partners you need fewer customers, but while the returns are slower, they are still plentiful enough and your enemies are fewer.

A few months later, another friend of mine, Antonio, whom I had known for many years, asked me if I knew of anyone in my circle of influence that may be interested in some weed. Well, call it naivety or curiosity, but I went back to him to ask a few more questions. It was during this time that I pondered how I might make a little part-time money on the side, on top of my casual wages.

Having already been given an introduction, I began dabbling in the art and science of raising plants indoors, learning to grow the plants from babies to mothers in around four months, and I became quite good at it. After I got over the excitement and fear, my 'horticultural venture' began to blossom and reap dividends. I dabbled in this enterprise for a couple of years.

I wasn't doing it to become a millionaire or a 'geezer' (Cockney slang for a 'well to do' individual), I actually got a buzz from having multiple sources of income and mixing with a large cross-section of people from all backgrounds, and cultures. Oh, and of course an immediate benefit was that my own personal weed was very cheap and effective.

Growing and selling the 'weed' was an easy way to earn extra cash on a part time basis through the laws of leverage, and by utilizing business partners without physically being present. Also, I believed weed was less harmful to others health wise, in comparison to many other recreational drugs available in modern day circulation.

One of the biggest joys for me was when I'd make 'hash cake.' I'd take it to work or parties and share it with all my friends for free, which contributed to endless energy, silly jokes and hours upon hours of rolling around in laughter.

But as time went on, I started to become a little bit obsessed with my part-time hobby, to the point where Jude expressed a number of times that I cared more about 'those little green babies' than I did about my own family, which in a way was sort of right.

Growing marijuana was never an easy pastime as paranoia was ever present. We would panic whenever we heard knocks at our door, especially during harvest time. We had a sunroom at the front of our house, where my indoor nursery lived. In this location the crop could be easily seen from the street had it not been for a thin black covering sheet. But to be honest, it wasn't the people knocking that worried me as most of my customers were friends.

My main worry was the strong stench the plants would give off during their last growing cycle, or blooming season. The strong and immediately identifiable odour would waft all the way through the house and into the street, which put both myself and my family at considerable risk. So I thought, enough was enough, and after a couple of seasons, I eventually quit the business.

I knew it was wrong and against the law. I didn't want to get caught, face a conviction and possibly time in prison, which would bring shame onto myself or my family. But, what started off as a bit of fun and an adrenaline rush, quickly spiraled out of control and took me down what I recognized to be the wrong path, especially in the eyes of God.

Even though as a child I was forced to attend church by my parents until the age of 16, I wasn't a 'born again Christian' throughout my involvement with marijuana. It wasn't until I turned 33 years of age that I felt compelled to go back to church and give my heart to Jesus. At this stage my wife had previously been going to church for about a year. In fact, it was her church attendance that helped change my mind, to start anew and leave my corrupt and illegal lifestyle behind.

Years later I understood that my journey as a Christian was about being a lot more considerate in my decision making. As a result I've become much more sensitive to others and aware of how my actions could possibly affect people, particularly my immediate family.

It was Antonio who first showed me how to turn marijuana into a business and we became very good friends over a ten year period, but like many friendships we lost contact at times.

I knew he had a girlfriend who was a heroin addict, unknown to Antonio at first. He bought three properties in Mackay over a period of three years and kept urging me to take my family up there and live, as the lifestyle was one of tranquillity and money apparently went a lot further.

Antonio had a sharp wit and very entrepreneurial in his way of thinking. He was constantly coming up with ideas and trends, which were ahead of our current era. For example, he suggested gourmet pizza takeaways and tapas bars years before they took off in Australia.

But, after he moved to Mackay from Bondi his personality slowly changed as his relationship with his girlfriend significantly affected his personality. We would chat on the phone and he would share with me his issues about his relationship, such as her always taking her handbag to the toilet whether they were out socially or at home. He didn't click that she was shooting up. She manipulated him into selling his properties one by one, obviously feeding him lies to fuel her addiction.

Over a period of five years, he became more sensitive, unhappy and introverted, spending too much time indoors, struggling to get out of bed and drinking alcohol daily to try and numb his reality. Then he was clinically diagnosed with depression and anxiety, for which he was issued medication.

I did my best to encourage and lift his spirits up. I talked a lot about God and I constantly prayed for him on the phone and asked friends to pray for his salvation as well. He even came back to Sydney for work, but during the six months he was here, we never actually saw him. He would make up excuses whenever we invited him over to our house.

When another friend broke the news of his death last year, my family and I went into shock, disbelief and then guilt. I wondered if I had done enough, said enough and prayed enough to help him through his situation. Each time I reflected on our friendship the tears would well up during quiet moments. Even now as I am writing this by myself, I am crying, the tears just keep coming. I've used too many tissues.

I knew he had a checkered past, but none of us are perfect and we've all done and said things we regret. However, in his last years he tried so hard to make up for his mistakes by working on Botany Wharf as a crane operator, then onto buying and selling property before finally labouring for builders.

What is particularly upsetting is when a person has such unlimited potential, a loving heart plus a charismatic nature, then they are prematurely taken. To me they still have parts of their jigsaw puzzle to finish. My faith is always tested after losing such close friends and family, but I hang on to my beliefs that one day in Heaven there will be tears of joy when we are able to hug and laugh upon meeting again.

Festive Season

TREATMENT 2

Before I knew it, that festive time of the year was upon us and my family and other close relatives decided to hold our Christmas party early this year, due to a few members going overseas to spend their Christmas in New Zealand.

Christmas is a time to reflect on the story of Jesus and his birth into our world. His birth signifies unification for families and loved ones to usually come together and celebrate their love for one another. Although Jesus was born a Jew, he showed love for everyone, for all races and for all classes of society, and Jude and I always tried to emulate his spiritual philosophy.

On this occasion we had a great day, consumed great quantities, indulged in delicious food, chatted amongst each other and some even took a power nap on the day. Even though I felt a little tired throughout the day, it was relatively trouble free with no obvious side-effects making a visit.

When Monday rolled around I went back to work on a later shift, but I started off a bit dodgy again, not feeling good at all. The nausea decided to make an appearance a few times especially in the morning, but luckily not with too much intensity. But, after a pizza lunch that day, I hit a wall of fatigue and was barely able to stand up. I really struggled for what seemed like hours. I forced myself to drink a few glasses of coke, in order to give me a caffeine boost.

It must have worked as I recovered to a point where I felt fine the rest of the afternoon. I left work for home, but when it got to 8pm my stomach started giving me problems, followed by indigestion. By the time I went to bed I wasn't feeling at all comfortable and I spent a restless night.

The next few days came and went without too much fuss, but the end of the week turned out to be an absolute shocker. Smells of any kind would send me dry retching, I couldn't even eat breakfast. I felt so terribly sick I just couldn't go in to work. This all happened before 5.30am, so I returned to bed until 10am, sick and fatigued. The rest of the day I drifted in and out of nausea, delirium and general sickness. My sense of smell was extremely heightened and made me feel very laid up.

The intensity of the medication this time around seemed much stronger than the last treatment, which seemingly had lulled me into a false sense of security. At times I felt my heart was beating out of my chest whenever I walked around or did any movement at all. Sweat was on my brow at most times. I often took my temperature, but mostly registered a normal 360.

I had to force myself to eat small meals. I recall once consuming a jacket potato, a salmon sushi, and a small portion of trifle across the whole day. Compared with my regular days this was a very lean eating schedule indeed.

The entire rest of that week were all very challenging days for me. Each day I battled nausea, sickness, and fatigue. Even though I worked throughout, there were periods during every day that I longed for home or the comfort of my own bed. Although, I doubt I would have felt comfortable even there.

Much more worrying was that my weight had dropped again by another two kilograms (about 4.5 pounds). Furthermore, new side-effects began to expose themselves, the first of which was a loss of hair. My loss of hair was first visible down below, followed by the scalp and then a distinct lack of facial hair, which included my beard, eyebrows and eyelashes.

My fingertips lost total sensitivity in all but my little fingers. I would get heart palpitations after climbing stairs and while trying to sleep. My left hip, where I'd had the bone marrow extraction, gave me more grief and kept me awake for hours on end. I wasn't allowed to take aspirin and anti-inflammatory medication whilst receiving treatment, and I didn't want to become a daily pill-popper, but had to resort to painkillers to remain sane.

In Europe the Christmas season and cold weather is normally accompanied by frost, sludge and possibly even snow on the ground. But the houses are decorated with holly and mistletoe, which is normally hanging overhead when you approach the front door. So whoever is welcome to your home is greeted with a kiss.

In England, the vibe is quite traditional and on Christmas day, the kitchen table is normally laden with roast turkey served with chipolatas, wrapped in bacon and bread sauce; baked ham, with a fruit crust; roasted potatoes, roast vegetables including brussels sprouts. For dessert some sweet mince fruit pies; Christmas pudding with custard; and to finish off are brandy snaps filled with berries and lemon cream. Port or sherries are traditionally offered as after dinner liquors.

What an absolute feast, I always missed the traditional English Christmas, although I did have a personal bent against brussels sprouts. In fact, I only know one other person who likes brussels sprouts. I know they are a very nutritious vegetable, but I'm not quite sure why they are so popular at Christmas.

Our landlords and dear friends Joseph and Paula had flown home to the UK to be with their family this week, and were having a lovely time experiencing a frosty English Christmas. This was of course a very different experience to what we were going through in Sydney.

Joseph and Paula were always very generous towards me and my family and insisted that during the time I was off work without pay, our rent would be reduced, so we had one less thing to worry about, a very very kind and considerate gesture.

My employers were also extremely considerate and allowed me to take a period of leave without pay until I was fit and well enough to resume work. But, they also paid me right through the Christmas holidays like any regular employee on holiday.

We had known Joseph and Paula since they emigrated to Australia around 2006. They have such a lovely family and own a Rhodesian Ridgeback for a pet dog, who is adorable. Their house had a two-bedroomed self-contained apartment upstairs, which they kindly offered us to rent off them at a very affordable price.

But enough fantasizing about Old England, because as it turned out, Christmas Day that year was a really good day for me. I could eat anything I wanted including prawns, oysters, baked ham, chicken, salad, and I was able to drink water without wanting to vomit. But, this was my last day of 'food freedom' for some time and I dreaded the next day and the thought of being zapped again.

I spent the rest of that day chilling and even went to the movies to see 'The Hobbit', which was so entertaining with very cleverly done combat scenes. Although Jude, Michelle, who was a friend of a friend and myself paid the 3D price and watched the trailers in 3D, the main movie was in 2D, which to me was very disappointing. I thought to myself the experience was a bit like life, mostly a fun ride with some very low points thrown in.

CHAPTER 6

A Poison Chalice

Who is Hodgkin?

Apparently this disease was named after the English physician Thomas Hodgkin, who first described abnormalities in the lymph system in 1832. The symptoms of Hodgkin's Lymphoma are swelling of the Lymph nodes, and although usually painless it often becomes painful in the armpits, neck and groin region. Other symptoms that became obvious to me were: heavy sweating especially at night; sudden weight loss with no obvious explanation; coughing or breathlessness; loss of appetite; fatigue and lack of energy; high temperatures that come and go; and a generalized itching and body rash.

According to the Leukaemia foundation each year in Australia around 550 to 600 people are diagnosed with Hodgkin's Lymphoma and approximately 100,000 worldwide, although it occurs more frequently in males than females. Overall it is a rare disease accounting for only 0.5 % of cancers diagnosed.

The exact cause of HL is unknown, but theories suggest that alterations in the lymph including a weakened immune system, an inherited immune deficiency disease, HIV infection and perhaps drugs taken to prevent rejection of a transplanted organ could all be factors. HL is treated by chemotherapy, a combination of radiation and chemotherapy or stem cell transplant if it has relapsed. Long-term effects can include fertility problems, a higher risk of developing secondary cancers in life, cardiac gut problems and damage to the lungs.

Going through this life-threatening journey I wanted to understand more about Hodgkin's Lymphoma and so I undertook to research the causes, and possible successful treatments. I found an interesting study by Mt Sinai School of Medicine in New York, in regard to toxins. Their work identified a total of 167 hazardous compounds in the blood and urine of adults (with an average of 91 per person tested) including 76 known to cause cancer, 94 that are toxic to the nervous system, 82 that damage the lungs, 86 that affect the hormone function and 79 that cause birth defects.

Alternatives

I was pretty much feeling OK for the first few days of Treatment 2, and I unexpectedly slept through the first few nights, which up till then had become a rare occurrence. Then I started on a new natural supplement called Zeolite, which was introduced to us through Jude's cousin, Dean. Dean is a very switched on person who thinks creatively, and always outside the box.

Dean's father Wally was diagnosed with throat cancer a couple of years ago, which was a shock to us all. His throat actually turned black. Wally had one treatment of chemotherapy and decided not to undergo anymore. Then he started taking Zeolite as a supplement and after just a few months his throat had improved. The result was not only fantastic, it was apparently tremendously successful.

The improvement was a very surprising result for a number of reasons. First, Wally had turned his back on traditional medicine at a time when his health was critical. Secondly, everyone was overjoyed that during this process Wally didn't suffer or experience any side-effects whilst taking this supplement. Dean was so overwhelmed that his father had progressed through taking this supplement that he naturally shared it with a lot of friends.

What this supplement apparently does is to trap and remove toxic metals, such as lead, arsenic and mercury that may have accumulated in our system through taking in toxins from the air we breathe or through foods in our diet. Then after trapping them it helps remove them, leaving essential minerals such as calcium, magnesium and phosphorous in the body. By reducing the body's toxic load, Zeolite makes the liver's job easier and therefore takes the strain off this vital detoxification organ, which then leads to a healthier liver.

Zeolite also helps to balance blood sugar levels, blood pH levels and enhances the immune system. Dean gave me this supplement to use in a drop form, which my body could tolerate. Another supplement I found useful was 'Vital Greens', which was introduced to me by a friend named Sean, a successful personal trainer who had been using it for the previous 12 months to help balance body pH levels.

Vital Greens is a nutrient and enzyme-rich complete super food which contains 76 nutrients essential to deliver optimal health, energy and vitality to every cell in the body. This product has certified organic ingredients, the correct ratio of minerals and trace elements, maximum absorption and bioavailability of nutrients in this form compared to tablets and capsules. Vital Greens optimise the acid/alkaline balance and being real food that's alive instead of synthetically made vitamin pills, it enhances intestinal health and is a source of essential amino foods, essential fatty acids (Omega 3 and Omega 6) and digestive enzymes.

I'm quite sure that by being involved in the fitness industry you must have an open mind to understand improvements in human physiology, and as such you are also exposed to information on supplements and the latest wonder concoctions. Being the friend he is, Sean gave me a two kilogram container at no cost and strongly urged me to use it. However, I really struggled to consume this supplement because it had to be mixed with water and each time I drank it, I was nauseous and often vomited.

I found out that pH levels in the body of 6.9 and below are conducive to disease. The optimum pH of your body should be slightly alkaline and range between 7.35 and 7.45, which is the level that Zeolite tends to establish. So I began to use both of these products as a daily supplement to maintain a proper pH balance, minimize bacteria, fungi, yeast and viruses and other diseases, which thrive in an acidic environment.

During this time I received an email about lemons and its many uses for bettering our lifestyle. The source of the information was fascinating and came from one of the largest drug manufacturers in the world. The lemon tree is renowned for its varieties, which can be eaten and used in a multitude of different ways and purposes.

We can eat the pulp, press juice, prepare drinks, sorbets, pastries, desserts and marinades etc. Most interesting is the effect it produces on cysts and tumours. Some say it is very useful in all variants of cancer and considered as an anti-microbial spectrum against internal parasites and worms. It regulates blood pressure, combats stress and nervous disorders, so it was worth a try.

So, with the permission of my doctor, I embarked upon a little bit of 'alternative' to match the 'traditional' treatments I was being exposed to.

Side Effects

TREATMENT 3

Today I underwent the next level of treatment on my unknown journey and the side-effects began to kick in straight away. I became terribly sick almost immediately after this cycle finished. That evening I had no appetite whatsoever so I went to bed early without any dinner and struggled to sleep.

The next morning began with dry retching, sickness then vomiting and this cycle continued for the next three days. Smells, fragrances, scents and food odours all contributed to the nausea and my continued throwing up. Odours from the following things were most distinctive in setting me off:

- Mangoes, (normally one of my favourite summer fruits).
- Lynx shower gel and deodorant.
- Taking a sip of normal drinking water.
- Walking into the bathroom or even past it.
- Any body deodorants whatsoever.
- People, especially with bad breath.
- Hanging styled deodorisers used in cars.
- Any body odour whatsoever.
- Lady's perfume of any brand.
- Cocoa butter body lotion (which up to now I used daily).
- Even my very mild aftershave balm.

My mental state of mind also began to feel the pressure this time around and I would become nauseous at particular times and places, but especially when: I thought about my chemo treatment; I spoke any positive affirmations regarding my health; I entered the hospital, even if it was just for an appointment; or if I was asked how my treatment was going.

I would feel sick just from waking up in the morning. My internal body clock would go off at approximately 6am when I would vomit and feel much worse for wear. If I ate a piece of toast I'd get severe stomach cramps for at least half an hour. This routine usually continued throughout the day. The only time I left the house was for a walk down the road. The fresh air was a nice distraction, the change of scenery was uplifting, but I still felt very sick with frequent bouts of dry retching and stomach cramp when I seemingly tried to do almost anything.

I even felt nauseous when I prayed for relief from my sickness or for support from God. I cried out to God to help me overcome these hideous reactions to my body, mind and spirit, and the following scripture came to me one day on the way to the hospital.

Trust in the Lord with all your heart and lean not on your understanding; in all your ways acknowledge him and he will make your paths straight.

Do not be wise in your own eyes fear the Lord and shun evil. This will bring health to your body and nourishment to your bones.

Proverbs 3:5-7

Perseverance

In what rapidly became a normal routine, I began each day with vomiting and nausea, but on one particular day I thought deeply about, and empathised with the plight of pregnant women. Now, of course I wasn't a lady who was about to give birth, but I know that most women go through a period of 'morning sickness'. Apparently this morning sickness can last anywhere from days to months through the first few months of pregnancy. During this period of the pregnancy the morning sickness can be tough, really really tough.

However, I identified whenever I saw or thought about pregnant women who were going through their nausea and sickness just as I was. I felt that people needed to pay tribute to pregnant women who suffered quietly compared to men like myself, who when sick felt that the world was about to end. Maybe I felt this way because I wasn't used to being ill, I didn't normally become sick very often and I was used to feeling jubilant on most days. Well that's my excuse anyway!

I was definitely feeling well below par, but being the festive season Jude and I arranged to hold a barbecue lunch for a few acquaintances including our close friends Reuben and Tracey, who have a very cute set of twins called Isaac and Elijah. This was to be our last social engagement with this lovely couple as they were about to move to Darwin to embark upon a new phase in their lives. Jude and I both knew we would miss them tremendously.

By the time lunch came around my appetite was still poor. On this day I managed to eat a small jacket potato with pineapple and cheese, a small piece of 'scotch fillet' with salad, and two flavoured ice blocks. Another one of my friends by the name of Joe brought along a box of 12 Krispy Kreme doughnuts. But do you know, I couldn't stomach even one doughnut, which was so incredibly unusual for me!

Later on we went to visit some other friends John and Chrissie, who were also a lovely couple and had recently given birth to a beautiful baby boy. We'd known them for over ten years and only seven days previously they had brought their son named Zane, into the world. He was a lovely little boy with a full crop of hair already. I struggled for energy throughout this day and didn't feel at all well, but it was so refreshing to get out of the house even for just a few hours.

By this time it was New Year's Eve and yet another set of friends, Pete and Sherina, made us some homemade pizzas for dinner, which was very thoughtful of them. The pizzas looked amazing, piled with toppings and even though I only had two small pieces we really enjoyed them. That night Jude, my daughter Tahlia and I attended a barbecue at yet another of Jude's friends' homes. Kate and Jeff were a couple that we'd also known for many years. Jude and Kate used to work in retail together at the same shop and each year we made a habit of catching up usually around Christmas time.

But in what was a real surprise this time around, Jeff and Kate really turned it on with an Asian noodle salad, chicken wings and pork spare ribs. I was feeling a little better and my appetite perked up somewhat so I ate as though I hadn't eaten for months. Well, in fact that was absolutely true as during this time my appetite had taken a vacation.

Unlike many countries and cultures around the world, we in Australia are able to eat and drink whatever we choose in abundance with no restrictions. So to round off the string of Christmas and New Year social engagements, that night I drank two bottles of non-alcoholic malt beer, two cans of lemonade, four cups of water and two glasses of wine. It was experiences like this that made me really appreciate the simple things we take for granted every day.

I recall when Jude and I travelled to Fiji for a holiday. Our package included an all you can eat daily breakfast and dinner buffet plus free soft drinks and wine. Back and forth we went at each sitting until we could eat no more. We feasted to the point that we could hardly walk back to our hotel room. After a few nights of this routine we sat back and observed the behaviour of the vacationers who had bought the same package and reflected on how amusing it must look to the local Fijians.

Coming from Australia where there is an abundance as far as eating and drinking is concerned, to a beautiful exotic third world island, you wouldn't think Australians would have the 'eat everything' attitude like 'pigs in a pen' just because they bought an 'all you can eat' food and beverage package. Being involved in treatment for a life-threatening cancer did often bring such thoughts to mind.

The next day was New Year's Day. Happy New Year! That day the weather was great, I felt great and amazingly I'd made it into 2013. To celebrate the occasion, my wife, daughter and I felt like doing something different. Maybe a drive to some place different and fun. But I was then overcome with nausea for which I immediately took some medication.

Each time I felt my nausea was about to start, I was advised to take a Zoffran (Ondancetron) tablet to combat the sickness before it kicked in fully, then I was advised to lie down for a little while to wait for the wave to pass over my body. Otherwise the nausea would suppress my entire body, and by then it was too late for any medication to come to my rescue. Sometimes this would work, but on many occasions it didn't. This is what I did on this particular New Year's Day, followed by a 30 minute power nap and then finally and thankfully, I felt good to go.

Still undecided about our destination we initially headed south, then drove to Bowral, a sleepy town just 90 minutes south-west of Sydney. It took quite a while, but we eventually sat down to a late lunch at a local cafe called Janek. Being the New Year's Day holiday it was the only cafe that was open, which meant it was very busy. But, after waiting 35 minutes in the heat the food was definitely worth waiting for. We ate a homemade hamburger, salmon and chicken panini with freshly squeezed juices and homemade desserts between the three of us.

The traffic to Bowral and back flowed easily and by 6:30pm, the time of our return, the day was still very warm. On arriving home our rarely used pool seemed to invite us in for a refreshing dip. It was a lovely way to end a lovely day. This was a day I'd term a top day, which I enjoyed immensely and despite my troubles I thought to myself, 'how lucky I was to be be alive and well, and loved.'

> *"Do you not know? Have you not heard? The LORD is the everlasting God, the Creator of the ends of the earth. He will not grow tired or weary, and his understanding no-one can fathom. He gives strength to the weary and increases the power of the weak. Even youths grow tired and weary, and young men stumble and fall; but those who hope in the LORD will renew their strength. They will soar on wings like eagles; they will run and not grow weary, they will walk and not be faint."*
>
> *Isaiah 40:28-31*

Over the next few days I recognized the development of a new and recurring pattern taking place. After waking up I would initially feel fine, but then within an hour I'd feel a terrible nausea with dry retching and lethargy. I was also on an emotional roller-coaster, feeling sorry for myself, moody, miserable, wishing I could fast-track into the end of February when all my treatments would hopefully be completed.

At this time however, I noticed my body starting to do things that added to my distress. I found that my hair wasn't growing back on my head, face or chest, which really didn't bother me, especially the latter. However, most worryingly my tongue and the ends of my fingers had developed black marks. Even though my taste buds had deserted me, my tongue still felt sore whenever I ate. The sensitivity at the ends of my fingertips had gone and they just kept tingling. My body seemed to be overheating with beads of sweat constantly on my brow. Water would normally quench my thirst, but now I couldn't stand the taste of it. Instead I had to consume cordial, juices, carbonated drinks and fruit flavoured ice blocks, which was all I could do to replenish my fluids. As for my appetite, three children sized meals were all I could manage. I felt like 'Benjamin Button' in the food department, decreasing in years as I got older. On the plus side throughout these days, we were saving a bit of money on groceries.

Even though I began to feel better and my anti-nausea tablets had reduced to just one a day, my fitness level dropped away severely. I had no desire to undertake any resistance training, push-ups or make the effort to train at the gym. This was particularly abnormal for me as my weekly routine included regular exercise. The only workout I was able to do was a 20 minute bike ride at medium pace and a few laps of the downstairs pool.

Due to my lethargic state I took an opportunity to take a trip down memory lane by listening to Reggae and R&B hits from the eighties and nineties, which I found to be so very relaxing. I had forgotten how much I enjoyed listening to music, uninterrupted for hours at a time as I'd done in my youth.

I recalled that whilst in my early twenties a few friends and I would spend hours and hours in the local record shop previewing tracks. A 'record' shop back then was well before the age of compact discs, which have now morphed again into mp3 computer files. I used to listen to the latest dance tunes on usually very much sought after and independently labelled records.

My friends and I spent years going to clubs and following the top DJ's around London's throbbing dance scene. Don't get me wrong, we weren't groupies, we were just like 'Billy Elliot' and loved to do nothing more than dance. We were the ones who stood near the speakers and danced and danced all night long, battling with each other and busting into new moves. In hindsight, I realize now where my tinnitus stems from.

Coming back to my present situation, and in keeping my musical tradition, I felt that I handled my sufferings better if I locked myself onto 'You Tube' and spent literally hours listening to music, one track after the other. It was a sanctuary for me and one that I never grew tired of. Music really picked me up, always! But please don't get me started on my favorite hobby or I won't ever finish this journal!

In the evening we responded to yet another invitation when Jude and I visited our friends Bill, Helen and Bessie for dinner, dessert and a catch up. These occasions became invaluable distractions for me and at this dinner we all had a great time and enjoyed great company.

CHAPTER 7

Descending

Gratitude

During our lives, I wonder how many of us actually stop and think of how grateful we should be for what we receive every day. I gave this some thought and compiled the following short list of what we are blessed with:

- The opportunity to be healthy on any given day.
- The choice of eating any food, at any time all year round.
- The support and care of good friends.
- The reliability of family when the going gets tough.
- Family whom we don't choose but are ours regardless.
- The ability to travel to almost any country, at the drop of a hat.
- The comfort of traveling without worrying if we will enjoy it.
- And then there is music... music... music!

I recall once watching a documentary whilst I was still in High School. It was about a young boy who had to endure his entire day and night confined inside a bubble, which became his whole entire world. The bubble had been designed within his parents' home as he had developed a condition which would kill him if he came into contact with the air we all readily and normally breathe every day to survive. In order for his parents to enter into his world, they would have to wear protective clothing from head to foot. Even if they just wanted to give him a hug or a cuddle, which is a daily requirement between all parents and their children. The young boy was under the age of eight years old, had lots of toys, games and entertaining devices to keep him occupied, but no friends his age to share, experience, wrestle, argue, laugh or play with.

Now before anybody starts feeling too sorry or teary-eyed for him, I'll also never forget the great big smile on his face as he played, rolled over and over again inside his bubble. The documentary showed how his parents loved and adored him so much, but they were the ones who were doing it tough, it was they that suffered and cried on camera throughout the interview. They were the ones who longed to be able to hug their son or have him in their bed all the way through the night. They were the ones who missed having their son living in their world with them.

Having now contracted Hodgkin's Lymphoma, in some ways I felt that I too was living in a bubble of sorts, cut off from life. But I felt eternally grateful and a deep and overwhelming sense of appreciation for the life I'd been able to lead to date.

*And hope does not disappoint us
because GOD has poured out his love
into our hearts by the holy spirit
whom he has given to us*

Romans 5:5-6

The Weather

It was by now mid-summer in Australia and this day was the hottest day of the year as the thermometer climbed past 41 degrees. There was some breeze, but the wind blew hot air and the heat lasted all day and into the night. In fact even at 2 am the temperature was still at 34 degrees. In our house, we had the overhead fans running continually just to try and circulate the air.

I recall that I spoke to my younger sister in the UK on that day because it was her birthday and the topic of weather was certainly mentioned more than a few times. I couldn't help mentioning the weather as the difference in seasons begs a reference to what the relative temperatures were on the other side of the world. If we were all back in the UK, with the freezing temperatures like they experiencing I'm sure that talking about warmer places would be the topic on everyones mind.

Back in England of course, it would be classed as a heat wave if the temperature were anywhere near 30 degrees. Breaking news..."31 degrees...Hottest February on record since 1966!" You see, the British don't actually know what real 'heat' is until they've experienced the over 40's in Australia. But my sister's reply to all of this was simply... "We shouldn't complain". It was statements like these that bolstered me considerably against the life-threatening adversary I was now facing.

My memories as a juvenile growing up in the UK were always of the summer months. Long summer days spent picking blackberries and strawberries and making our own sweet lemonade from freshly picked lemons. Or embarking upon long walks and adventures with my brother and sister, Michael and Julia. We could be gone all day until 8pm in the evening or even later at night before our parents would start to be concerned. These were the days before mobile phones were invented and parents just couldn't keep track of where their kids were at any given time. As I entered the next stage of my life I increasingly began to hang out with friends and I discovered music, bought clothes and experienced the enjoyment of travel.

These days, whenever I go to the UK with my family from Australia, even though we have a great time experiencing the history, food, travel, culture and just spending time with my English family,

I can't help but notice how dark and grey the sky is most of the time. Outside of its very short summer, England is mostly cold, overcast and wet, and this definitely affects your overall mood.

Upon reflection, I find that as we get older, life becomes less complicated and much more simple to understand. But the environmental factors over which we have absolutely no control can have a very powerful hold over us. The weather definitely plays an important part in determining our daily mood and forming our attitudes to life.

Freefalling

It was around this period, halfway through my third treatment that I really reached a low point. Runners get it during the final gruelling stages of a marathon. Inexperienced players sometimes get it when the opposing team takes the lead in the grand-final with ten minutes to the final whistle. With an overload of assignments to complete just before their final exams, students can also get it. But it's completely different when it involves your health and I very nearly lost the plot.

People could say…"but Joseph where's your faith, you've been a Christian for over ten years, why don't you pray, or read your bible." The fact was that my energy was completely sapped; my mental faculties weren't working in unison with the rest of my body. I wasn't eating, the chemotherapy drugs were really kicking in, and medication I'd been prescribed wasn't counteracting anything.

Even though I developed a bad case of cabin fever, just stepping out of my house for fresh air brought on acute paranoia. I felt as though everyone was staring at me, my clothes were just hanging off my now bony frame, and I felt that my identity was completely gone.

I often thought to myself that… "conversation with a close friend would be great right now." Then tears would well up in my eyes. They were tears of anger, frustration, embarrassment, hopelessness, endless pain and suffering... and they just continued to flow. I felt like I was going to burst with despair.

I whispered to myself, God why don't you take me now, to a land of milk and honey, where there will be no more despair, anguish, struggling and sickness. Let me go now. Visions of close friends and family I had lost to death engulfed me. My spirit felt crushed and I could feel myself descending into a hollow and empty space... an abyss.

I quite quickly got myself into a psychological state that had to be addressed. I wondered if this was how Robinson Crusoe felt before making friends with animals, or whether I should be having full blown conversations with a football companion like Tom Hanks' friend 'Wilson' from the movie Castaway? The slight difference was that I wasn't on a desert island, and I was lucky in that I had good friends, as well as a close biological and church family that would contact me on a regular basis.

During these 'black' episodes, my one penetrating thought was who would look after my family, Jesse, Shannon and Tahlia as I had no legacy for them to ease their own lives if I died now! Under these circumstances, Jude and myself had so far avoided the drama of having a will drawn up, let alone deciding who would get what.

I knew I had to snap out of this depressing state. The negative thoughts were going on and on, but the 'self-pity party' had to stop somewhere! So I made a determined effort to move on and move up. I heard a voice say to me... "Shake it off Joseph, Shake it off now!"

"Joseph, Shake it Off" I heard again. "Stop being so selfish, grow up and face this problem like a man!"

The reality of the moment hit me like a ton of bricks. I realized it wasn't time for me to go yet, there was much more for me to do, more for me to be, much more for me to live for. I had two strong reasons to continue... the first was, of course, consideration for my family, but oddly the second compelling reason to fight every day became the completion of this book. I felt my book had to be completed mostly to help others going through this indescribable experience. I felt this experience had to be communicated to the rest of the world and that provided me with the will and courage to fight on.

PET Scan

Unfortunately, the persistence of the illness kept wearing down and me and just when I was starting to feel a little better my sickness and nausea kicked in yet again. I found myself having to take anti-nausea tablets more frequently and feeling overwhelmingly sorry for myself once again. I really didn't know if I could cope with more chemo treatments than the six to eight I was already on. The way forward depended solely on the results of my PET scan.

An MRI or CT scan can give us excellent photographs of different parts of the body to identify enlarged nodes or tumour masses, however, it's difficult to tell if a lump or mass has tumour cells in it only by measuring its size and shape. But a PET scan can measure the activity of the mass and can be used for staging or mapping the disease. The PET scan helps to decide what kind of treatment is appropriate and shows whether a lump on a CT scan has cancer or not. They told me that a PET scan had the same effect on the patient as undergoing an X-ray, but the escape of the radiotherapists into their lead cladded room to turn on the machine says it all!

Before undergoing a PET scan you can eat up to six hours prior to the procedure, but you cannot engage in any strenuous physical activity. It sounded to me like the advice a coach would give to an Olympic athlete before their big event.

A small amount of radioactive material is then injected into your body an hour before the scan is performed. The scan itself lasts for approximately one hour during which the patient has to lie as still as possible the whole time. Listening to music to help one relax is fine, but reading books or magazines was definitely out. I wasn't surprised about this at all, as the amount of gossip in Women's magazines would send anybody's pulse racing.

Some people have chemotherapy treatments for six months at a time. Some have multiple cycles of chemotherapy. Let me state right here and now that it takes guts and determination to soldier on through those times and I developed a great admiration for the suffering of people having to go through the nightmare of multiple chemotherapy cycles. I grew to hate it with a passion as any normal person would.

I only had to start thinking about my next treatment to bring on dry retching. As mentioned already, by this time my appetite was non-existent, and I had lost the desire, vision and my zest for life. I found myself really struggling with the side-effects of the chemotherapy. But I often recalled a 'Tupac' song and kept repeating it over and over in my head.

> "Baby don't cry, I hope you gotcha head up
> Even when the road is hard, never give up
> Baby don't cry, gotta keep your head up
> Even though the road is hard, never give up!"

I began most days like a Zombie. I felt like I was on an open field which stretched for miles. The air was full of dense, heavy fog. There was no clarity, no vision, no visibility, no sound. Just me, staggering and swaying around like a drunkard, lost in a void of emptiness. I was utterly and completely alone.

I was totally depressed at the prospect of having to undergo my upcoming fourth chemotherapy treatment and was in no mood for idle chat with anyone. Even catching up with close friends had its struggles. At the hospital, I couldn't bear the thought of socializing with other patients or even striking up conversations with staff. I felt numb, lethargic, sick, non-productive and I had an overwhelming urge to skip the treatment completely and return home.

Throughout the treatments, my close friends and family would ring me up, encourage me and generally want to know how I was doing. They'd send scriptures by text message to help me push through the suffering and meditate upon. Most of the time the effort it took for me to string a few sentences together was huge and absolutely exhausting. After a chemo session I'd leave the hospital a physical wreck, I'd have to be driven home and I'd simply sleep for what seemed like hours and hours. But events like going through cancer treatment teach us that life goes on and it's left to us to make decisions as to whether to sit in doom and gloom or get on with life as best we can.

I remember that Jude had a few work friends and their partners come over for a South American style bar-b-q one evening. Somehow I was able to sum up the effort to sit and socialize for the evening. Despite what I'd been through that day and even though I could only hold down a little of the food, the evening was fun, it passed the time and the event somewhat lifted my spirits. I just couldn't get excited about the Chilean-Argentinian style feast, which normally would have been delicious to my sense of smell and taste.

Somewhere in the midst of this journey, I had a prodigious craving for comfort food in the form of Kentucky Fried Chicken. This was peculiar for me as I hardly ever enjoyed a meal from that particular fast food outlet. We would visit our local KFC only ever about twice per year. Anyway, on this day I bought a piece of chicken, carefully unwrapped it and placed it in my mouth, but then felt the biggest disappointment. It was a funny feeling as my taste buds had gone on vacation and there was utterly no taste whatsoever. I gave the meal to my family and walked away with my head down thinking to myself "what a waste of time that was!"

CHAPTER 8

Taking A Break

My Birthday

I was between treatments when my 46th birthday arrived halfway through January, but it came at the wrong time health-wise as this day turned out to be the absolute worst day of the year for me so far. Yes, you guessed it. I woke up with my old friend nausea, some vomiting and I was in a foul mood for the entire day. Both physically and mentally I felt lethargic, I couldn't focus at all and the intensity of the side-effects were three times what I had experienced so far. Because of how I felt I couldn't even answer my phone.

It was a 'shocker', with bells on! For those who don't know what that means, it's an English term for 'couldn't possibly be any worse!' The malaise and numbness lasted all that day and into the next. Even though I was very grateful for family and friends wishing me Happy Birthday, my spirit was completely broken.

As I've already mentioned, Jude and I are of Maori and African heritage and our traditions are centered on large families, friends and friends of friends always being around. A birthday will usually be celebrated with a gathering of some kind, no matter what age that person is turning. It's the occasion and not the number that brings the family together. We would always celebrate birthdays, and not just our own as the backyard in the house before Malabar with its outdoor kitchen facility was a fantastic entertaining area. Consequently we also used to invite many friends around to celebrate their birthdays at our place.

So here I was, aged just 46 years old, but feeling like a broken down grumpy old man. I often thought of my hopeless situation and talked to myself. It was like staring into a reflection pool and I was watching the way my life had turned out.

"Let's face it, I'm no spring chicken, I now require eight hours of sleep as a daily minimum, and when my wife and I go to social events which pass midnight, it takes me two days to get over it. Even on a lazy Sunday afternoon I find myself wanting a 'nanna nap', unless my favourite rugby league team, the South Sydney Rabbitohs are playing."

"During the winter months, I normally wrap myself up in a jacket and scarf, not to be fashionable, but because of the amount of weight lost I now more easily became very cold. I asked myself 'how can younger guys sport t-shirts and shorts... don't they ever feel the cold?' If I accidentally cut or bruised myself, the healing process seemed to take weeks. It took me years to finally come to the conclusion that I was no longer bulletproof and invincible, rather I was just an old fart."

So how would I answer if someone asked me 'how old I was and what I did for a living'?

All I could say was, "Well I...", "umm, well I'm in my mid forties, and I work 40 hard hours a week as a chef. My work is based on a seven day roster, which usually means that I work on alternate Saturdays, so two out of four weekends every month are spent working. What's more, I'm just working for someone and don't manage or yet own my own business."

Now I know quite a few friends of similar age to myself, who turn up for work, have coffee for half an hour, punch out a bit of work then morning tea for 45 minutes, punch out some more work, take an hour and a half for lunch, see a couple of their existing clients over a cappuccino, make some calls to line up tomorrow's prospective clients, then go home, and they were pulling in six figure incomes!

Other friends I know are given a base sales quota, but would have the option to work from home most of the time. They only need to turn up at head office for one day per week if at all, then fill in the rest of their time cold or warm calling. As long as they satisfied their monthly quota at their own pace, they were otherwise left alone.

You couldn't find this kind of freedom however in my job, oh no, it was always go, go, go until lunch time, then go, go, go again until knock off time. I don't want or need sympathy here, as I know we all have a choice to decide how we should earn our income, I'm just simply telling you what my world at this time was like.

Whilst my younger days were spent in spontaneity and constant adventure, routine was now how I lived my life unless we were away on holidays. I was also becoming a victim of envy especially whenever I pulled up at traffic lights and glanced across at a really prestigious or expensive car. After seeing how young the driver often was, I'd immediately pass judgement in my mind about how lucky these young guys were, that their family could let them roam around in such luxurious cars.

So today I should have been celebrating my 46th birthday with family and friends, in reality apart from my wife and daughter, I had the toilet bowl, vomiting and only self-pity for company. Happy Birthday Joseph!

But today of all days, my birthday was not going to be one of those fun, out of control, family fun days. The highlight of my 46th birthday was to be able to make a short walk down the road with

Jude. Malabar is a lovely place for a stroll, and a great place to clear your head and think without too many people around or traffic congestion. I just had to get out for a change of scenery and some fresh air, but as if things couldn't get any worse, we got soaked by a downpour in the process.

A Hub Of Activity

If any person ever arrived at our home with social phobias, they would have been totally rehabilitated by the time they left. Our boys Shannon now 25 and Jesse aged 27 would often have their mates around our home, usually at weekends, sometimes even for warm-up drinks and food, before they headed out for the evening. Sometimes people came over just to hang out and enjoy the nibbles that were always on offer.

We were also a host family for overseas students studying English. Often for six months at a time we would accommodate two students in our home and they became just like members of our family. We were a loving and friendly host family for about ten years and treated all the students fairly. We hosted Chinese, Japanese, Ukrainian and Colombian students, and they were all usually cordial, very nice in fact and mostly always polite.

We did have one experience however, that we will never forget. It was when we had some short-stay students, who came for just two weeks. One particular young woman from China was memorably horrible, which was unusual as most people from China were fabulous. On her very first night she was totally obnoxious and had a bad attitude towards everything and everyone. On the second night she started taking out her frustrations and becoming quite angry at our playful daughter, who was just five years old at the time.

Jude couldn't stand by and watch her rudeness so she jumped right in and gave it to her. An immediate and emotive argument erupted, and I knew that if it continued, Jude would lose her cool completely, so the other male student and I quickly stepped in to break it up. We then immediately informed the students' Homestay agency of what had happened and we demanded that the student be transferred that night. The agency asked us to work it out for the rest of the week, but the situation was unretrievable. So we had to refuse the request and in the end they quickly moved her out. Jude was quite rightly hopping mad over the whole affair!

Back then our home was like a boarding house with people coming and going all the time. It was fun, exciting and very busy as you never knew who was arriving or what was going to happen next. However, we have since downsized from a seven bedroomed home to a two bedroomed apartment and our sons now live independently with their friends, so you could say that our home has become a lot quieter.

Even in relaxing, tranquil surroundings I found that to be able to converse for more than one minute was just too much of an effort. Jude always remained very supportive and empathetic towards me. She was my 'Rock of Gibraltar' and I'll be forever grateful for the patience she always showed towards me especially when I felt unable to socialise.

The next five days were all similar in the way of nausea, sickness, diarrhea, lethargy and the entirely new experience of multiple stomach cramps. I was in a bad way and didn't really feel like talking to anyone at all. My friend Alex from Darwin called during this time and I recollect that even while on the phone with him I was dry retching as I strained to converse. By this time I'd known Alex for nearly 20 years and he had become one of my very closest friends.

During the past few years however, he had hit rock bottom. He had his heart broken when his longtime girlfriend split up with him and returned to England. He also lost a few of his investment properties due to market fluctuations and some poor decision making. As time went on I noticed that he also lost his self-respect and dignity as well.

Alex would want to talk when he was going through his darkest moments and I always did my very best to encourage him and try to lift his spirits. However, even though much grumbling left my lips, it was definitely a struggle on this occasion. By conversations end we both felt sufficiently inspired to carry on over what we both knew would be challenging days ahead. I can't emphasize how important such seemingly small encounters were, in helping me to contend with difficulties and the enormity of what I was facing.

During this most debilitating of weeks I tried to drink plenty of fluids, but couldn't stomach much more than toast, dry biscuits and tinned spaghetti in the way of solid foods.

During this time I was affected by what I called, 'the saliva experience'. When my mouth wasn't active, meaning that it wasn't chewing, eating or talking, it would fill up with saliva, causing me to spit frequently. If I went to sleep without a lolly in my mouth, I'd have to get up and spit constantly throughout the night. It sounds disgusting doesn't it? Well, it was that and more!

With excess water accumulating in my bladder due to the intensity of the medication, saliva would frequently run from my mouth. I had turned into the 'dribbler'! I was consistently excusing myself to run to the bathroom when we had company present. It was embarrassing, awkward and uncomfortable and seemingly carried on for months. The oncology nurse at the clinic told me this happens when the body is dehydrated and requires more fluids.

It was at this time that I remembered a close friend of ours called Teah, who was dying of cancer. When we visited her during the last few weeks of her life, the very same mouth thing was going on with her. She always had some tissues in her hand to spit out whatever fluids were in her mouth and tragically died soon after. It was a very frightening and confronting memory.

Time Out

I was feeling much better this morning and decided to go to the Powerhouse Technological Museum with another close friend called Sam. His daughter Sarah and my daughter Tahlia, who are exactly the same age, also joined us.

It was a hot day and on the way there in the car my stomach started to turn, the sweat began to drip off my brow, and the ever-present nausea kicked in. My daughter asked if I wanted to turn the car around and go home, but I thought it would soon pass. Well, it didn't, the nausea lasted for most of our day there despite trying everything in my power to muster the strength to stay with it. I told Sam later that I just wanted to flake out on one of the Museum benches and wait for it to pass. He was very understanding. Indeed everyone seemed to understand and showed me much empathy. Despite feeling so poorly I didn't want to be a party pooper because it would have meant that Tahlia, Sarah and Sam would've had to find some other means of entertainment for that day.

Despite the day's ups and downs I surprised myself by going the distance throughout the Museum visit and this very slight improvement was significant as I only had to take one anti-nausea tablet that day. My specialist gave me free reign to have what I needed (within limits) and three anti-nausea tablets were my normal daily dose.

The next night we were invited to a very special double 40th birthday of one of Jude's cousins Kiwa, who was sharing the big occasion with his wife Ness. Adding to the big night was their wedding anniversary, which was also being celebrated at the same time. It was a really pleasant occasion. They had a three-piece band playing, and the food and drinks were fully catered for. There were around 30 guests including Jude's other cousins, the group being all around the same age bracket, between late 30's and early 40's. The theme for the evening was 'seventies' and everyone dressed up accordingly. There were many memorable highlights of the night, but when one of Jude's cousins missed their steps and took a tumble on the dance floor, the whole place erupted in laughter. She wasn't drinking either, which made it even funnier. The atmosphere was one of fun and happiness for the rest of the evening.

I'd finished work just before Christmas and was told not to return until I felt better, but my position was always open. However, I didn't return until well into April, which happened to coincide with the end of Treatment Two.

Spending so much time at home, the scene became so monotonous and overwhelmingly boring. I would switch between the bedroom and lounge room for a change of scenery, and the bathroom for throwing up. Most of my days of late had been spent in my bedroom sleeping fitfully. So Jude, Tahlia and I decided to drive to The Entrance on the New South Wales Central Coast for a short break, as I had some vouchers from the Novotel. We thought it would be a great idea to take a break from normal everyday life for a few days. Also it was the school holidays and I knew Tahlia needed some time-out from watching me feel sorry for myself day in and day out.

The Entrance is only 90 minutes by car from Sydney, north along the beautiful New South Wales coast. On arrival we had a late lunch, did a bit of window shopping and went to the supermarket to buy some essentials to last us during our stay. We went on walks, ate out for all our lunch and dinners. It was a lovely break from the normal day-to-day activities as we relaxed in the spa baths and spa pools and did absolutely no cooking whatsoever. It gave the whole family an opportunity to unwind, with great weather to top it off.

One of the highlights of those few special days was when Jude and I revisited the venue where we were married 16 years previously. The property had a lovely outdoor setting and we both thanked god for these wonderful and treasured moments.

> *And we know that God causes all things to work together for good to those who love God, to those who are called according to His purpose.*
>
> Romans 8v28.

CHAPTER 9

Restless & Rocky

Support

I was now in my mid forties and basically, still a plodder. I lacked savvy knowledge as far as financial security goes, so reliance on my week-to-week pay was crucial. As a family we still had to pay the school fees of which we were always behind. Our Visa credit card payments were in arrears. Car insurance and utility payments kept pouring in, and of courses food and a plethora of other general bills always needed attention.

I was also aware of my new dependence on the family and felt I needed to contribute in any way possible to take the economic weight off Jude's shoulders. At this time Jude was working two different jobs and coming home absolutely shattered every night. We were definitely experiencing financial hardship, but didn't want our daughter Tahlia, to know about it. Rather, we wanted her to feel secure, throughout my sickness. She was always very helpful, but didn't really understand in too much depth what was going on in our household. Given the difficult circumstances of not being able to perform paid work through my sickness and provide for my family, I made a call for support.

Not being able to tap into any other source of support, I thought I'd take the initiative and contact CentreLink. This body is the Australian welfare agency that temporarily supports people experiencing financial difficulty. I didn't feel any shame in doing this as I'd been paying taxes into the system for years. I reasoned that even if they couldn't contribute direct financial support, they may be able to provide some guidance as to what I could do to help relieve the growing burden, as I was always conscious of not letting my family down.

Unfortunately, my initial approach to CentreLink was received by a suspicious officer over the phone. The person at the other end of the phone made me feel as if I was trying to wrought the system, and I was most upset by the way I was treated. Not being able to work was not a personal choice, I had been gripped by a life-threatening illness.

I was required to verify my identification and hand in a form for a family payment. When I visited the office I had to stand in a queue for over an hour before I was able to speak with a consultant. Then after all that, they had to schedule another appointment for me to speak with another specialist consultant, so all I could do that day was to simply hand in my forms, which took another 90 minutes.

My actual appointment lasted just two minutes, and I had the temerity to ask why the initial desk consultant couldn't perform this simple procedure. Why couldn't I have handed in my documents to them, to save a considerable amount of time, but I was abruptly told that " you have to follow the protocol".

I personally felt this experience highlighted a real waste of time and resources, but fortunately I could access my emails, play games and access the internet on my mobile phone while waiting. To pass the time I thought that I might get lucky and witness some incident. I hoped perhaps a bitter and irate person who felt the world owed them a living, might enter Centrelink and cause an uproar with the staff.

I always found these kind of people entertaining in such circumstances and 'people watching' was one of my favorite hobbies. This was how I occupied myself during that long boring wait at Centrelink. Luckily the poor overworked staff weren't required to deal with any unreasonable customers that day.

At the end of the day, after a long, long wait and after furnishing letterheads from my medical specialists verifying my condition, there was a breakthrough. I eventually qualified for the maximum support payment of just $80 per fortnight, but it was something and always thoroughly appreciated. The small payment was primarily because my wife Jude earned over the minimum threshold for people in such circumstances.

That night, Jude and I caught up with a few close friends for dinner. I really looked forward to this evening as it might cheer me up. We went to a place called Danny's Seafood Restaurant. It turned out to be a very stormy night, so the restaurant was not as busy as it normally would have been. However our spirits were not dampened and we were determined to enjoy the evening.

There were two musicians playing the guitar, going from table to table entertaining and asking what requests people would like to hear. They were very friendly, professional and became a highlight of our night. On the menu was an assortment of fresh and fried seafood and our meals were both wholesome and tasty. Our friend Joseph brought a bottle of Sake that became a perfect accompaniment to our food. My doctor had placed no restrictions upon me for consuming alcohol and mostly I had no desire for it, but on this night I didn't hold back. Generally, it was a fun night with good friends and great entertainment.

Later that night however, became a rocky and restless one for me. I wasn't surprised as such feelings were becoming the norm, but I didn't know if it was the alcohol, the meal or just my depleted self.

I woke the next day feeling very 'dodgy', and I couldn't help saying to myself "here we go, nausea city here I come again". If I had to rate myself on how I felt out of 10 throughout that day, it would have been as follows.

From - 7am to 11am - 6 from 10.
From - 11am to 2pm - 4 from 10.
From - 2pm to 5pm - 2 from 10 (Uggh!).

As usual I became worse as the day progressed. Even though we often caught up with friends over dinner, I never consumed more than half a glass of wine, and most of the time alcohol never touched my lips. Since my teenage years I had always refrained from drinking and preferred juice, whilst my mates drank alcohol. The taste of beer and spirits never really appealed to me.

There was nothing that distinguished the next day from any other except that I spent the afternoon looking at juicers at the Moore Park SupaCenta with Jude and Tahlia. Later on, Kiri and Bruce, Jude's cousins from Padstow dropped in for a social visit. We didn't ever see many of them, but it was good catching up for a couple of hours and very nice of them to show their concern. They explained that they were in the area and wanted to pay us a visit and offer their encouragement.

I distinctly recall that this day was particularly delightful, so in the evening Jude and I decided to take a leisurely stroll around Malabar and the beach. It definitely wasn't a power walk, but within half an hour after arriving home, I plummeted again. On reflection, I was definitely pushing myself too much and too early.

Spring and autumn were my two favourite seasons because the weather was mostly just perfect. Although these periods were changeable with cool breezes and occasional warm spells, I generally felt much more uncomfortable in the depths of a hot and humid summer, which was always just t-shirts and shorts. Whereas it can get just too damn cold in winter and you must always dress warm.

Another lovely day again, not too warm and not too cool, so I thought that on such an especially beautiful spring morning, I'd try to walk from Coogee to Clovelly, a distance of some three to four kilometres. I wanted to see if the way I fell apart yesterday was just a one-off event. Besides, it killed an hour of my free time, which was in plentiful supply at the moment.

I finally reached home about 3.30pm and had pushed myself for almost 60 minutes. However, just 30 minutes later I felt my inner bodily workings, my immune system, my good cells, my bad cells, in fact my whole body shook with pain. A very familiar routine came back into play again and it took me down memory lane to that place of diminishing hope. That place, where I felt like I wasn't ever going to beat this invader in my body. I don't usually swear, but on this occasion I felt so bitter and dejected that I expressed my anger and frustration in a long string of four letter words.

I remember one particular day the cancer nurse gave me a follow-up call to see how my health was progressing. It made me realise that there must certainly be many patients who find themselves undergoing very difficult experiences, and in this regard I wasn't alone. My personal battles were not only physically, but psychologically draining. So I always found the services provided by both the Leukaemia Support Group and the Cancer Group very supportive.

The financial and community support provided by these two groups really helped to buffer the blows I was constantly being dealt at this time. I was always very grateful for the support of my family, friends, my church and work communities. Whether it was a simple text message, a phone call, financial donations, general good deeds or a simple prayer, it was always very welcome. All these expressions were demonstrations of encouragement and love at this very difficult time, and I honestly don't know how I would have handled myself if I had been alone with no support network whatsoever.

Pleading

TREATMENT 4

On this day I asked the nurse if I could have a one week extension of time before my next chemotherapy treatment, explaining that I just wasn't handling the situation too well and psychologically I felt I wasn't recovering. Of course the nurse had to ask her supervisor, who in turn passed me on to another supervisor, who came to speak to me and must have called the shots.

I slowly became annoyed as, yet another person asked me a series of questions. I wasn't as if I was trying to do a runner from the scene of a crime, I just pleaded for an extra week. Eventually my haematologist Dr. Susan had to be notified. The final answer that came back from her was an emphatic yes, but it was a difficult process to go through. I guess they thought it would be harder for me to complete all my cycles if I delayed the program. Also, rearranging their already planned appointments and schedules proved to be most troublesome, especially if other patients did the same thing.

It was 'cyclone season' up north and the news reported storms smashing into Queensland, New South Wales, the Solomon Islands and parts of the United States, but my personal storm somehow went unreported. If you ask anyone who knows me well, they'd tell you that I was usually virus-free all year round, and if I did catch anything it normally only held on for around 24 hours. But over the next few days I felt like a prisoner in my very own world.

Despite being given a respite from chemo, I first caught a cold, which was followed by a debilitating bout of diarrhea. I developed a runny nose, coughed frequently and experienced persistent headaches. I restricted myself to home and just one or two necessary trips in the car. During this time my eyelashes and eyebrows also decided that they would go on strike and as a result, they completely disappeared. I would wake up with sleep in my eyes and a constant frown due to the bright sun.

You probably know this, but I will mention it anyhow. Apart from being useful as a beauty accessory, I found out that eyelashes protect our eyes from dirt and dust. They also let us know when a foreign object is headed toward our eyes by quickly sending a message to shut our eyelids. Just like the sensitive hairs inside our nose that create 'boogers' and help to trap dirt and germs before they get inside and bother our lungs. I thought how glad I was that our eyes have lashes and not boogers hanging above them!

The following days all seemed to run into each other with similarities that were difficult to decipher. Jude and Tahlia started fasting and restricted their diet to anything grown from a plant or seed, but no dairy, meat, fish or sugar was allowed. On the other hand, although nothing had changed in my diet, each day I experienced an episode of either vomiting or diarrhea. My nausea had just started to fade away and I began to feel as if I was getting back to a level of normality, when my appetite again took a huge nose-dive.

For me, living a normal life meant that I could eat whenever I was hungry; perform physical activity without feeling nauseated afterwards; go anywhere and do anything without worrying if I was overdoing it; occupy myself with anything to last the whole day. It was a very depressing and unwanted change in my life that forced me to sit around being sick for most of everyday.

I normally prefer to feel tired or fatigued at bedtime too, not sitting up wide awake in the early hours of the morning. Adding to the boredom was the fact that we had no cable television, which meant no television during the early hours when I couldn't sleep.

I found my days were now being taken up mostly by spending endless hours waiting around at the hospital, CentreLink, or the doctor's surgery. I was always aware that having to frequent these places was beneficial to my ongoing struggle, but they weren't the most uplifting venues to be around.

I had to postpone my last chemo treatment twice due to my severe ill-health. To be honest, I found myself increasingly questioning the benefit of having to endure all the pain and even whether I wanted to go through with the treatments. I'd been so unwell for so long now that I began focusing on my low points, which was brought on by the nausea, the stomach upsets, the general sickness, the diarrhea, my anticipation vomits and never being able to be my normal everyday Joseph.

I knew it wasn't the right attitude to combat this affliction, but I was being 100% honest with myself. The truth was that at no stage was I ever asked whether I had endured enough! My doctors always just carried on with their day to day business without too much emotional investment in my individual case. My frequent visits helped me to understand this unemotional approach as I watched other patients become severely ill. Focusing on the task at hand was the doctor's best defence in dealing with what often became their own emotional distress at seeing some patients deteriorate and submit to their fate. I unfortunately now had just too much time to think on what my life had become.

CHAPTER 10

Overwhelmed

The Depths

It was the day after we returned from The Entrance that I had an appointment with my specialist, Dr. Susan regarding my progress to date. I'd certainly been through a lot by this point and was holding my breath for some sign of hope, or just a little good news would do. Just before I left for our holiday, both an MRI and a PET scan were performed on my body and I was about to receive the results.

Magnetic resonance imaging (MRI) is a scan used for a medical imaging procedure. It uses a magnetic field and radio waves to take pictures inside the body. It is especially helpful to collect pictures of soft tissue such as organs and muscles that don't show up on x-ray examinations.

So here I was in front of Dr. MacCallum waiting for the inevitable. What could she possibly tell me this time? Susan sat me down and gave me a long sympathetic stare. We've all heard the term 'death by chocolate,' well here's a new one to suit this situation, 'death by Chemo'! If the Lymphoma wasn't going to kill me then the treatment was certainly heading that way.

All kinds of thoughts were racing through my head; what if I had to go through another six cycles of chemotherapy to make absolutely sure we'd zapped the cancer, or maybe another six months. Or, much worse still, what if Dr. MacCallum said, "Sorry... its not working... you will need a stem cell operation because your stem cells have taken a battering due to the high doses of chemotherapy".

Was I about to experience what most people don't like talking about? The old saying, "there are only two things guaranteed in life, death and taxes", which paints a very gloomy perspective of life for us. Is there any wonder why the majority of the population view life through a pessimistic lens.

From an early age everyone learns to fear death and most deaths occur unexpectedly when we least expect it, catching us off guard. But some people know ahead of time when their death will occur. When diagnosed ahead of time, terminal illnesses allow a person to place their affairs in order, forgive all the people who we feel may have wronged us, solve any conflict and relationships and say goodbye to loved ones and those close to us.

When faced with death many turn to religion or faith to answer their own questions about the afterlife and eternity. There are those who say that they went to heaven or hell and then can't wait to share their testimony with as many people possible. As a born again Christian I believe when we die that our soul goes to heaven and then we start a life of eternity without pain and suffering. A good friend of mine Steve passed away about four years ago. As his love for God deepened during his last few years, he repeated to me on numerous occasions, "I'm getting closer, it won't be long now Joey, before I go home!" The expression on his face said it all, as he laid in his casket on his funeral day, so peaceful, ever so peaceful.

Now back to what Dr. MacCallum had to say to me, which I was determined not to allow it to shock or surprise me. It seemed the last couple of years was priming me for this very moment.

Dr. MacCallum announced that my Lymphoma had reduced 86% so far, which meant we were finally making progress! Phew, and phew again! That was the best news I'd been given in ages. The good news was quickly followed by a warning that I still needed to get through another two or maybe even three more intensive cycles of chemotherapy. I knew that despite the fact this was the first good news I'd had for months, my journey back to living a normal life still had a long way to go.

The night before going onto an even more intense fourth treatment, I could feel my body anticipating what it was about to go through. The nausea, vomiting and general overwhelming sickness. As I entered the hospital a shuddering started to develop from my head right down to my toes. I thought to myself "Thats great! I feel sick even before I've been given the treatment to make me sick!" That day our landlord and another good friend, who also went by the name of Joseph, was kind enough to pick me up, spend his time in the waiting room and bring me home. What an absolute champion!

I distinctly recall that it was 'Robert Burns' Day' that day. Robbie Burns was a loyal Scot whose best-known poems were Auld Lang Syne and Ode to a Haggis. Robbie Burns Supper is celebrated on January 25th, the tradition started 200 years ago in Scotland and Northern Ireland, then spread to the United Kingdom. Haggis is the traditional dish served at a Burns Supper and since moving to Australia in 1994 I hadn't come across, or eaten any haggis at all.

Burns suppers may be formal or informal, both typically include haggis, which is often drank with whisky. The Haggis consists of sheep's offal mixed with suet, spices, oatmeal, stock and seasoning, traditionally boiled in a bag made from the animals own stomach lining, nowadays often boiled in an artificial casing. We made a lovely haggis with mashed potatoes, with peas and carrots for the whole family. It was accompanied by a small sample of Rhubarb

Vodka, which was quite distinctive and tasty. Although I could only manage a wee dram, we all loved it.

Burns is the poppet of the common man. By eating humble food at a celebration rather than a grand elaborate feast, we celebrate the simplicity and humanity of the Scottish poet who was Robert Burns. Little did I know that this was going to be my last enjoyable meal for quite a while. My decision to stop work indefinitely after undergoing treatment two was definitely the right thing to do, as each treatment cycle thereafter knocked me for 'six', a cricket term for being hit out of the park!

Not Over Yet

TREATMENT 5

It was the middle of February 2014 and the first few days following a treatment were always the most gruelling, which pushed my mind games to the extreme. One minute I was Arthur, the next I was Martha. I use that terminology not because I was unaware of my gender, but because I was in a confused state of mind for most of the day, not knowing if I was going or coming and spending useless energy pacing back and forth.

I was really appreciative that my workplace bosses were so empathetic towards me. They continued to buzz me and check on my progress and told me to take as long as I needed to recover. The next few treatments were a critical part of my chemotherapy package (sounds special like a bumper pack, well it was, full of surprises). The daily struggles became both predictable and monotonous as my treatments now had more significance in killing off the cancerous cells. My body just surrendered to this chemical infusion as it slowly sapped my energy reserves.

Over the following days I quite naturally felt under the weather, lethargic, weak and generally miserable. I travelled to no more than three places: the toilet, the bedroom and the couch. On the fourth day the cancer nurse paid me a visit to check on how I was going.

By this time most of my senses had completely dropped away. My taste buds had once again become de-sensitized and I had no way of knowing if I was eating a bad meal or a good one. Some people might be happy to be in such a predicament (haha), but I found it very difficult to enjoy any meal that had no taste.

I've heard people say that chemotherapy kills everything in the body thats living, but whilst trying to sleep either in the night or during daytime naps, I kept recalling memories from my past. Especially in the way of school friends, people I went to college with, my associates and friends from when I was in my teens. I remembered names, places I visited, and minute details of the events I attended. Although a little strange, as far as I was concerned, chemotherapy was an amazing memory aid as these flashbacks came from as long as 30 years ago. I can recall that LSD had almost the same effect on me, although this was of course was when I was trying to find adventure in my early teens.

In regard to my outward appearance, some side-effects became painfully obvious. The hair on my scalp was growing in a Mohawk fashion, with short straight hair. My beard was patchy and grew very slowly, and shaving only had to be performed twice a week for one minute each time. My eyebrows were thinning, fragrances, odours and smells were greatly enhanced, and even my eyesight had deteriorated.

But returning to the visit of my cancer nurse who gave me some anti-nausea injections and put me on a drip for approximately an hour. The health authorities' contribution to the community was extremely helpful and a great service for chemotherapy patients such as myself, who could be treated out of hospital.

However, on this occasion I had trouble sitting down after she left, and I found that standing or lying down for more than five minutes at a time was extraordinarily difficult. I paced the floor of our home back and forth, upstairs and downstairs and felt I was going a little bit potty. Tahlia my daughter asked if I was OK, but I couldn't give her a yes or no answer. Was it paranoia, anxiety or was I on my final descent? My heart started beating louder and faster. This disturbing episode went on for a couple of hours.

Then these debilitating feelings abruptly stopped. I found myself comparing my circumstances to a kitten with a minute needle stuck in its tail, racing up, down and around, indecisive or incapable to pull it out or leave it alone. I found out later that I was allergic to one of the medications the nurse had given me, which was responsible for the onset of an anxiety attack. We now know it was the medication called Maxalon, which turned the next few days into a complete blur.

I became increasingly worried, scared and dubious of ever getting up and walking around again. Most of my time during this phase was spent in either a sitting, kneeling or laying in a horizontal position. Whenever I did walk around it only lasted a few minutes before the sickness and nausea would again make itself felt. The experience was one that left me absolutely exhausted. However, our mind is such a powerful tool that can be used to either propel us forward, or prevent us from moving on.

Today was no exception in the way of challenges, plus it was Tahlia's first day of school after having had six weeks on holiday. Although most of her time was spent looking after her dad through observation, caring and love, I still had to drop her off and pick her up from school because she finished at midday. But, despite a sense of disorientation I managed to complete these simple chores and also visit the chemist to pick up some medication, without dropping to my knees or the couch for safety.

These very simple tasks left me zapped of energy, and the hot weather just added another difficult element for me to cope with, as it was 26 degrees and sunny. When it was hot, my condition became more challenging, my body temperature rose, I sweated profusely, my muscles seemed to shrink and my whole being turned into a lethargic mass.

I felt like Ray Charles without the music prowess, skills and talent. The reason I felt like him was nothing to do with his career and what made him famous, it was more the fact that even on cloudy days, I had to protect my eyes from the daytime glare by always wearing shades. Whether I was in the house or not it was another indication that pointed to how sensitive my outer shell had become.

I still had four weeks before I was required to return to work in May 2014, but I constantly wondered whether I'd be fit enough to do so. I wondered too, whether I'd ever make it out of this endless gloomy tunnel. My life seemed to be slowly slipping away and everything began to feel so distant to me. But, I often thought about how so many others before me had endured cancer and this made me more determined to overcome this affliction. I believed even more, that "what your mind can conceive and believe, you can achieve!"

It was about this time that I began to feel awareness of an inner strength building within me, and what's more... I knew where it came from. Whenever I felt I had hit rock bottom, I was being pulled up spiritually from the depths of my despair by reading a poignant verse of the bible.

In the day when I cried Thou answered me, and strengthened me with strength in my soul."

Psalm 138:3

CHAPTER 11

Faith & Love

Beautiful Jude

All the way through this excruciating ordeal, my beautiful Jude was mentally and emotionally very strong, although physically exhausted most of the time. There was never any talk of the inevitable, or what was next for her and the family if I didn't make it through. I guess even though her faith was severely tested it remained steadfast throughout, and she always had the rock-solid attitude that everything would be all right at the end of the day.

We went to visit Jude's cousin Dean and his wife Ness at their family home as he was not only a member of the family, but works as a financial advisor. We talked about Life Insurance and planning for eventualities if the worst scenario played out. For me this informal semi-social visit quickly became a reality-check that in the event I died from the cancer, my family would still be able to cope financially. Although I'd given this scenario the odd casual thought from time to time, I'd never actually considered that my death was either a possible or probable outcome, and so having a third party address this scenario absolutely hit me like a ton of bricks!

But much more sobering was the effect this discussion had on Jude. When I glanced over at Jude from the corner of my eye, I could see the tears already welling up in her eyes. This was the first and the only time I ever noticed the effect that my troubles were having upon Jude and it thoroughly tore me to pieces. We both burst like an overfull dam into uncontrolled weeping. Then simultaneously reaching for the tissues that Ness had so strategically placed on the table, we gave each other the tightest hug for what seemed like an hour.

Dean and Ness then tactfully explained that taking this step wasn't scaremongering, but just sound planning, and that both him and Ness had already made arrangements in the unlikely event of their deaths. As responsible adults there was a lot to contemplate but we were, from that point on, able to talk openly about future eventualities and arrangements. Jude has already told me where she would like to be buried, back in New Zealand on her family plot. As for me... err... umm... I think a cremation would be my preference.

Valentine's Day

On a much brighter note, Valentine's Day, the day of love, was coming up very soon. I bought tickets for the movies so that Jude and I could see 'Les Miserables'. Then that very same evening, another set of friends invited us over for dinner. Some of their family had flown over for a little holiday from New Zealand and were leaving in a couple of days' time. Anyway, after much discussion as to the merits of either, we unfortunately had to cancel both engagements due to my seemingly endless indisposition.

Throughout the length of my treatment the following quote often came to mind: "If at first you don't succeed, try and try again." I lost count of the number of times those words went through my head, but they became somewhat of a mantra for me and popped into my head at my lowest moments. My social calendar was constantly being adjusted to compensate for the day to day fluctuations in my health, and nothing could ever be planned, that's for sure!

Valentine's Day eventually arrived, and it just so happened that Jude wasn't working that afternoon. So knowing that my disposition could turn at anytime, we decided on the spur of the moment to visit one of the local cafes in Malabar for brunch. We both selected a really tasty dish, which was accompanied by freshly squeezed juice. We enjoyed an uncomplicated but pleasant meal together and were able to celebrate our love for one another with a simple yet very meaningful Valentine's Day kiss.

I was somewhat surprised however, when the food came out as I couldn't help noticing that the brunch portions seemed to be unusually large. Maybe I just thought they were large because my appetite had dropped from six to just two small meals a day, which was enough food for a seven year old. Consequently, I was now looking at meal quantities through the eyes of a year two student.

Feeling unusually well, that day I travelled into the city to splurge on myself and purchase some training shoes from 'Espionage', who many regarded as the best athletic shoe shop in Sydney at the time. On my way home I picked up Tahlia from school and briefly called in to see my in-laws, John and Keriata. We were only there for 30 minutes or so, but as I stood up to leave I suddenly felt dizzy and overwhelmed. John and Keriata could see I wasn't myself and urged me to sit down and wait until I felt better. I waited 10 minutes, but the situation didn't improve, in fact it was getting worse.

I started to sweat profusely, then felt very anxious and uneasy. I felt totally bereft of energy and my head began swimming in circles, with my body wanting to go in one direction while my legs were going in the other. I raced to get to the bathroom, but didn't quite make it. All voluntary control of my body was lost and I ended up in the master bedroom, half on the bed, half kneeling on the floor. Keriata came in right behind me, but I was in a complete daze for what I thought was minutes. My out of control body shakily attempted to stand up and reach the bathroom, so I could vomit.

Unfortunately, I never quite made it and violently began throwing up on the carpet, and of all places, my in-laws bedroom. A thought flashed through my mind that what a wonderful opportunity this was for pay back if I had interfering in-laws or a troublesome mother-in-law, but that was never the case with John and Keriata. Fortunately there was a thick towel lying on the bed that Keriata quickly positioned for me, under my chin. After five minutes of chundering and two towels later, the spewing finally ceased.

Keriata placed a cold towel on my forehead to cool me down. I gradually became more conscious and slowly regained physical control of myself. I thanked my lucky stars that this latest episode didn't occur five minutes later, whilst I was driving home, or perhaps earlier that afternoon, whilst I was shopping. Such an incident would surely have ruined my street credibility in Espionage Footwear forever. In fact, it would have ruined my street credibility anywhere, full stop!

John and Keriata could see I wasn't myself and this is where I earned the nickname 'spaghetti legs', as my body went in a completely different direction from my legs! They could see my distress and very kindly brought Tahlia and myself home, then watched over me until Jude arrived home from work that night. I was very aware of what had happened and determined if possible not to repeat the incident as no one needed an encore performance of that day, but the nickname stuck and became a standing joke between all of us.

But whatever had gripped me continued to have its effect as I felt lethargic, cold and was running a fever by 9.30pm that night. When Jude arrived home she could see I was suffering and immediately took me into the emergency department at the Prince of Wales Hospital.

I remained under watch at the hospital for the next four and a half days attached to a drip, being constantly monitored and fed with fluid and oral antibiotics. I was placed in the intensive care ward (ICU) and on a number of occasions I'd just start sweating, felt out of control and would violently throw up, losing all bodily control in the process. Whenever this happened I'd hit the panic button and within 30 seconds a member of the medical team would come rushing in to my aid.

The ICU staff were fast and really professional. I knew one of these medical staff members through a mutual friend, his name was Richard and this little episode bought our personal relationship even closer.

However, on my second night in the hospital some of my family and a few close friends came to pray over me and anointed me with oil from Jerusalem. Yes, the oil came all the way from Jerusalem, which was a wonderful thing to do and lifted my spirits a great deal.

I wondered how one would obtain oil from the holy city of Jerusalem, and had a vision of it being transported by donkey courier. I imagined 'donkey courier post' written on the side of the box it arrived in. The oil was in a minute vase-like bottle with a screw twist lid. My well-wishers were only with me for 15 minutes, but I was truly grateful and humbled that they had taken the effort to visit me late at night. We prayed together:

> *The Lord is my shepherd I shall not want. He makes me lie down in green pastures, he leads me beside quiet waters, and he restores my soul. He guides me in paths of righteousness for his names sake. Even though I walk through the valley of the shadow of death, I fear no evil for you are with me, your rod and your staff they comfort me. You prepare a table before me in the presence of my enemies, you anoint my head with oil, and my cup overflows. Surely goodness and love will follow me all the days of my life, and I will dwell in the house of the Lord forever.*
>
> *Psalm 23*

Initially I thought I was recovering, but after a couple of days my body started responding to the antibiotics with nausea and diarrhea. The nursing staff gave me some additional medication to help me cope with it all, and I felt I was becoming an all consuming pill-popping machine. However, despite my weight having dropped 10 kg to 74 kg, and feeling a little sleep-deprived I gradually improved, and after my four and a half days of hospital care I was ready for home.

On the positive side, my daily visitors of course were the best of company. Jude was continually with me and my family and friends visited daily, which really lifted my spirits. I also had a room to myself during my time in hospital and I was fortunately able to order the deluxe TV pack. This included free to air TV, plus four movie channels that were aired all day and throughout the night, which was nice entertainment for me and helped pass the time considerably.

But during this four day hospital stint I was somewhat consumed by my thoughts. I understood that I had been in a dark place over the last few weeks. I was stubborn, difficult and negative toward myself. Confusion occupied my mind as I was unable to determine what was positive for my long term recovery and what actions I took that might have negative consequences. I could not see the wood for the trees as there was seemingly no way out of this mess. I asked myself the same question over and over.

"How could I take any more chemotherapy when I was in such dreadful health?'

Worry too had taken a firm hold over me. Dr. Charles Mayo, founder of the famous Mayo clinic said, "worrying affects the circulation, the heart, the glands and the whole nervous system. It profoundly affects your health. I have never known a person who died from overwork, but many who died from worry."

Over the last few weeks I had become ambivalent about the treatment, I doubted continuing with the program and even contemplated the inevitable. But after being bedridden for almost five days my thoughts slowly turned around.

After leaving hospital I had a day and night to prepare myself both mentally and physically for my final chemotherapy treatment. As if a light had been switched on, I reasoned that as I'd had 80% of the chemo already injected into my body over the last few months, what difference could another 20% make to ensure a cure of my HL disease?

I knew that worry brought on anxiety and that the beginning of anxiety was the end of faith. However, I could also see the other side of the coin, and understood that the beginning of true faith was the end of anxiety. In the end I had the good sense not to make big decisions when I was physically and emotionally unsettled. After psychologically battling with myself for what seemed like weeks, after persistent phone calls and much to my family's and friends' relief, I finally agreed to complete my last chemotherapy cycle. They all said the same thing. "Well Joseph, you've come this far, there's just one more treatment left."

I agreed, but thought to myself... "easy for them to say!"

Final Countdown

Having agreed with my haematologist to continue with the final chemo treatment, my resolve was tested again when I experienced a bout of heart palpitations. Previously, I had mentioned just after treatment number 2 that I was experiencing irregular heart beats and flutters. Well, ever since then they had refused to go away. It would become more obvious after walking up stairs, sitting down, when just relaxing or mainly after I laid my head on the pillow to go to sleep. At my relatively young age, heart problems were definitely new to me. Thoughts would race through my head like, "you'd better be careful, you're heading for a cardiac arrest". I entertained thoughts like,"heart palpitations happen to middle-aged men with bad diets and eating disorders". Then I'd take a trip down memory lane, remembering the British pop group Madness who released a weird video about a corporate executive who worked too hard and had a cardiac arrest.

These persistent thoughts got the better of me, so I mentioned it to Dr. Susan just before my final chemo treatment. She was always very much on the ball and immediately scheduled an appointment to see a cardiologist over the next few days.

After spending a bit of time with the cardiologist, answering a few questions, wearing a heart monitor for 24 hours, undergoing an ultrasound and running a battery of tests, his conclusion was that the chemo was not doing my heart any favours. He thought that my heart had been stressed by the treatment, but that it would heal.

He suggested that either I should have the chemo reduced, or not have any at all, and that he would make my specialist doctor aware of all we talked about. I was prescribed some medication and made an appointment to see him following my next PET scan in one month's time. But after a relatively short delay due to this cardiac scare I was finally given the green light to proceed.

TREATMENT 6

This was it! I was now able to begin the countdown toward the completion of my final chemo cycle. My father-in-law dropped me off and remained at the clinic to make sure I was deemed physically fit enough by the medical staff to have chemo that day. All the usual procedures were carried out and the treatment went ahead.

As I was an overnight patient for the first time, the chemo was administered to me in a hospital bed, which was pleasant and comfortable. After this treatment I was informed that I'd be given a saline solution through a drip, which apparently helps to flush everything through the various body tissues and organs. I was told earlier that the saline was a great help in reducing the side-effects.

If hospital beds were not so scarce and money wasn't a factor, I'd recommend that all chemo patients should receive this saline infusion after every cycle as it was very calming and left you in a relaxed state. By evening time, there were minimal staff on duty and the treatment room had emptied to just myself resting in a ward bed. It was very nice to have my own personal space and the communal television to myself for a little while.

Later on, another overnight patient came into the room to watch the television as well. We struck up a conversation and for the next three hours we chatted, laughed and swapped stories about our childhood and life back in England. His name was Tony and he came from Liverpool in the UK. He was what we in England call a 'Scouser', and Scousers are very energetic people with a great sense of humour. Well, I thought he made the perfect Scouser! He had also been through chemo three times himself and was now having a stem transplant.

I always thought I was doing it tough and there were many instances where I saw life through a negative lens. Here was someone who was much more positive, and yet had been through a much more physically and mentally challenging experience than I had. He was nearly 50 years of age and he mentioned that his life had been a very enjoyable one, but stated emphatically that if his cancer returned, he would have no more treatment. Tony inspired me to be more grateful for things we all take for granted in our everyday lives.

I thought to myself how… ''One man can be enthusiastic for 30 minutes, another for 30 days, but it's the man who is enthusiastic for 30 years who makes a success of his life.''

The next day I wished Tony the very best of luck with his personal battle and I then thankfully left the hospital. My in-laws, John and Keriata very kindly picked me up and dropped me back at my home. Deep down, I felt satisfied that the cycle had now been completed. Any lingering negative thoughts that had been at the back of my mind regarding the last cycle, had finally been put to rest.

Myself and the whole family were greatly relieved that I had finally completed what I hoped to be, the last chemotherapy cycle. Passing this milestone provided me with a major sense of accomplishment. I felt for all those children and adults who had ever battled any type of cancer and endured the treatment, as surely a great sense of relief floods over your entire being on the day you complete the last cycle. It was almost as if an imaginary certificate of achievement had been presented to you from the oncology team.

However, the 'show' as they say wasn't over yet. We all knew that my particular strain of cancer was very aggressive so further tests were needed to see if the chemo had completely eradicated the HL growth.

I tried very hard to be very mindful of the fact that at any stage my health could suddenly deteriorate, but I could't help looking ahead towards the future with some hope. This was the first time in four months that I could actually think about what lay ahead without shuddering and dry retching.

The next day I received a good seven or eight calls from family and friends. A few were wondering if I had completed my cycle and enquired about my long term prospects, while most were well-wishers bestowing me with their support and encouragement.

But I thought my health was going to get worse, perhaps much worse before things made a turn for the better. Even though I wasn't vomiting today, I found it difficult to speak fluently. I murmured and slurred most of my speech. It was as though my tongue was disjointed from my mouth, but that didn't matter anymore as all I had to do now was to endure!

CHAPTER 12

Glimmer Of Hope

The Light

One of the many calls of support I received came from a long time friend by the name of Richard. We had developed a habit of contacting each other quite regularly. However, over the previous six to nine months Richard really became very supportive and encouraged me a great deal throughout my weekly ups and downs. I found his words were always very powerful and particularly heartfelt.

On this day he mentioned how courageous I was for going through with the chemotherapy and he told me it took guts to endure such a treatment. Richard seemed to be able to time his supportive comments perfectly for when I was feeling especially vulnerable or emotionally weak, and I often felt tears welling up in my eyes during these conversations.

Deep down though, I knew it wasn't being courageous that made my tears flow. It was knowing that there were people out there who cared so dearly for me. I reflected that for most men, tears leave our eyes with great difficulty as we often tend to bottle up our feelings. Whereas, it's a well-known fact that females outlive males purely because they know how to release their emotional tension.

The next few days were a waiting game. If my body followed the pattern of my past five treatment cycles, I sort of expected to be hit with bouts of maximum intensity sickness and nausea. However, this surprisingly didn't happen. I did get the side-effects of the chemotherapy, but amazingly they seemed to occur on a much smaller scale.

This time around I was mentally much stronger and prepared to cope with what I knew would be coming my way. I believed that having being reduced somewhat, the chemo would have less of an effect on me. I convinced myself that my body would recover quicker due to the flushing of saline continually throughout my organs for 16 hours. But most of all my faith was now at its strongest.

All my family and friends were praying for my recovery and great results in my health. I knew prayer was a two-way communication with God. Praying always unburdened me from worry and stress and I knew God would help pull me through this final hurdle. However, when two or more people are gathered and praying for the same outcome, it becomes such a powerful instrument that only good comes of it. Prayer is what Jesus did continually throughout his life and particularly during his sacrifice.

Throughout my personal health crisis I regularly turned to the Bible, which is God's word and speaks the truth. The Bible never contradicts itself and is historically accurate. I wasn't the only believer as the Bible is the most sold book of all time and is regularly on various bestseller lists.

> *I urge all men first of all, that requests, prayers, intercession and thanksgiving be made for everyone, For Kings and all those in authority, that we may live peaceful and quiet lives in all godliness and holiness. This is good and pleases God our savior, who wants all men (and women) to be saved and to come to knowledge of the truth.*
>
> *1 Timothy 2*

In three weeks' time, I would be submitting myself to another PET scan to determine if the Hodgkin's Lymphoma Disease (HL) had been eradicated. However, I was still bothered by questions: "Would this be the end of the crisis? Had the series of treatments been effective? Would I need to undergo further treatment?" These questions filled my mind and I found myself reflecting on the disease and just how and why it picked me to be its host.

When I was diagnosed with HLD over two years ago I had radiation continuously for four weeks. Then I thankfully went into remission and the cancer stopped growing. It was during this time that I went looking for the cause of HLD in my body, and in general. But to my intense disappointment, I couldn't pinpoint an exact cause. I then began researching the disease and found that there were many causes that can trigger HLD.

It seems that stress turned out to be the biggest contributor, but how? A study in the British Medical Journal in 2004 estimated that 75% of cancers were caused by environmental and lifestyle factors. Another report by the Columbia University School of Public Health estimated that diet and toxins in the environment caused 95% of cancers. Even the air we breathe may be polluted from transport and air pollution.

Today's buildings are more airtight and well insulated than years ago making them vaults for germs, bacteria and chemical toxins. We are exposed to toxins and pesticides every day through our crops being sprayed, carcinogens building up in plastic bottles, unfiltered drinking water, cosmetics, air fresheners, animal fats, household cleaners, fish, dental amalgams, insulation in walls and ceilings, water pipes and heating ducts from the 1950's, amongst other causes.

Food additives, preservatives, bleaching agents, ripening agents and flavourings are also in excess and are detrimental to our long term health. Everything I've mentioned above causes different levels of stress either directly or indirectly. All these factors might seem like doom and gloom but, we can definitely assist our immune system from being bombarded with toxic chemicals by making sensible lifestyle choices.

Back On Track

By April 2014 and after four hard long months, I had finally completed my treatment, but still had to wait a few more weeks to get the results.

For lack of guidance a nation falls but many advisers make victory sure.

Proverbs: 11-14

The appetite that had deserted me over the last few months slowly began to creep back and I now began to feel hungry more often. Even though my meals were quite small, I started consuming four or five small snacks a day. Not only did this make me feel a little better, it triggered an alarm that our grocery bills might also be returning to where they used to be, and I might even begin to make social visits to our local butcher.

Earlier on in my writings, I mentioned that both Jude and Tahlia were eating healthier, cutting out dairy, excess sugar, meat and fish. Well that had now finished, so we had all decided to tailor our eating habits to incorporate the meat, fish and a small amount of dairy. I was also so appreciative that my taste buds returned to semi-normal from their little holiday, which enabled me to again enjoy the taste of food to its fullest.

To be honest, my sleeping habits at night had been non-existent for quite a while. I would go to bed between 11:30pm and 12:30am, wake up every couple of hours, toss and turn for 30 minutes then drift back off to sleep. I missed the routine of work, and the mental and physical stresses that tire our bodies to the point of wanting to and maintaining a good night's sleep.

People are creatures of habit and often get used to certain daily routines and customs. My mum used to bake turkey a specific way by adding brandy and orange peel. When asked why she added these ingredients, the answer was always the same "I'm not sure, but my mum used to do the same thing." So, what do you know, our Grandma did it as well, but no one ever asked how this intergenerational custom started.

One of my habits I never questioned was my compulsion to exercise and play sport, whenever I felt the urge. It was always something I really enjoyed. I represented my high school in rugby league, football and athletics and was always in the running relay team. I played in the local district rugby league team as well. Then went on to practice Karate for three years, joined the local boxing club, then started training in gyms to keep fit and body-build.

Also in the middle of my active teenage years, during the mid –eighties, 'Hip Hop' and 'Break Dancing' debuted around the world. A few friends and myself formed a dance group and danced first on the street, sometimes for money. Then we progressed to performing in clubs and on other occasions to promoting drink labels such as Bourbon, Malibu and Vodka etc. There were dance crews in quite a few cities with names like Connect 4, The Rock City Crew, Breaking Glass etc. For the lack of something more original we called ourselves 'Precinct 9', as there were actually nine of us.

Some of these street dance groups went on to become semiprofessional and even featured on television. Most people in the cities accepted this new dance trend, but it took more time in the regional areas. We found this out when we performed once at a venue in Yorkshire called Halifax. After our performance had finished a few lady's applauded, but the guys showed their appreciation by smashing a few glasses and advancing menacingly towards us. The place was pretty dodgy so that was our signal to make a quick exit. We told our promotion manager to make sure he checked out our future venues for personal safety and security before booking us. It was always an adventure and we had heaps of fun.

Whenever I was unable to do physical exercise for whatever reason, I felt strangely out of sorts. So two weeks after the final chemo treatment finished I was very glad to begin riding my bike and, once again hit the gym. I now felt confident enough to start a regular training routine beginning with light resistance training and gentle stretching. I took it easy to begin with, but it felt good to be getting physical again, even though my body took awhile to reacquaint itself with physical conditioning and the sweating that goes with it.

After my initial workout the inevitable DOMS set in. I think DOMS is an acronym in the exercise world for delayed onset muscle soreness. This can kick in one or two days after strenuous activities or exercises, and generally lasts for a few days. Having had no activity whatsoever for months my muscle soreness started after a couple of days and lasted for an entire week, during which time I was just too sore to continue with any kind of passive stretching.

On my last birthday I received a voucher from my sister-in-law and her husband, Donna and Andy. I decided that now was a good time to make use of it by booking an appointment for a massage. However, of all the massages I have ever had, this one had to be the most painful I can recall. As we all know, the benefits of a massage can improve our body systems and we usually feel great afterwards. However, the chemo treatment combined with my inactivity had taken a real toll on my body and it took another week for me to get over that massage.

By week three post final chemo I also thankfully began to lose my smell phobia. I sort of understood and identified with what dogs go through on a day-to-day basis. They can't go past a person or object without sniffing them all over. Although this was not what I chose to do during my illness, much to my annoyance, it was what my nasal alarm bells chose to do. How interesting the animal world is. What if it was normal for humans to act like dogs and urinate every ten minutes, up against all sorts of obstacles whilst out for a walk. Or, display crazed sniffing all over everyone you meet. It would be just like living a skit directly out of 'Monty Python'.

All joking aside however, as I gradually realised that my health was taking a turn for the better. My days were much more productive. My life did not revolve around staying at home and the hospital, anywhere near as much as in previous months, because I was now able to cope with a more extensive roster. If I were to describe my daily 'list of things to do' at this point, it would go something like this:

- Catching up socially with friends.
- Training at the gym and doing some exercises.
- Build my appetite for food.
- Consume more food on a regular basis.
- Reduce my mood swings (mostly visible to my wife, Jude)
- Improve my attention span, enabling me to focus.
- Work more on the computer.
- Spread jokes and laugh more heartily.

These were just simple everyday things which most of us regard as everyday living, but not everyone is able to do them. The last few months had shown me that my health had deteriorated to the point where I was incapable of performing the simplest of tasks, due to my precarious physical, mental and emotional state. There was a part in Martin Luther King's famous speech, which comes to mind and expresses my feelings perfectly.

"When we let freedom ring, when we let it ring from every village and every hamlet, from every state and every city. We will be able to speed up that day when all of God's children, black men and white men, Jews and Gentiles, Protestants and Catholics, will be able to join hands and sing in the words of the old Negro spiritual, Free at last! Free at last! Thank God Almighty, we are free at last."

Martin Luther King

I too, now felt 'free at last' from my life threatening burden and it felt so very good!!!!

It was now week four post chemo when I reflected that, having an occupation that you really loved from the heart, plus being able to earn a living from it, was for so many of us and definitely for myself, a dream vocation. So after what I'd gone through, just being able to return to work was an immense blessing.

This week I rolled up the sleeves and started back at work. It felt so good to be 'useful' again, to add purpose and structure to my life, to meet and converse with my work friends, and it was especially gratifying to start earning some money of my own again. Jude had provided mostly everything for me and the family during the difficult phases.

I often feel a passion burning inside me. You might call it my zest for life. Some days it fires up, other days circumstances get in the way and the flame burns lower almost to a flicker. I believe there is a special passion burning inside every one of us and we have a duty not to let it fizzle out. I see no point in getting to the end of our lives and then feel totally unfulfilled at the finishing line.

Searching deep down inside for things that make me passionate about life and then being able to use that as a contribution to society is important to me. Being able to help family, friends and others during their times of greatest need would be immensely satisfying and I feel I'm getting closer to this goal through having lived this experience. Fulfilling peoples' lives and perhaps even scratching a living from it is now a goal of mine.

Love, Hope & Faith

It was now the middle of May 2014, week five post chemo and I had a meeting scheduled with both my oncologist and hematologist. I expected to be updated about the latest results of my most recent MRI scan that I'd undergone. I was very apprehensive, but fairly upbeat and looking forward hopefully to finally hearing some positive results. I constantly played out in my mind what the conversation with my consulting doctor might be...

"Hello Mr Anaman. We have your results and we are pleased to tell you that they are negative. The lymphoma has been eliminated and will not be returning again, therefore no more treatment will be needed for you in the future, but we would like to do a routine check every six months. We are very glad to report that you are free of the disease." I was free at last!

Sadly, it didn't go the way I had imagined. Unfortunately clear cut, finite vision of throwing off the Hodgkin's Lymphoma was not to be. After I had undertaken the scans, I had to wait for two very long weeks of nail biting, sleepless nights and uncertainty. Then, I couldn't take the uncertainty any longer and decided to contact my doctors to enquire as to the results. Closure and an end to this misery was all I wanted.

Apparently, regardless of the result of the scans the specialists handling my case had already made up their minds about the next stage of treatment. Day surgery appointments were limited to mornings between 9am to 12noon, while my work hours ran from 6am to 3pm. This meant that I had to take two separate days off work, to see each specialist.

The good news, no, THE FANTASTIC, AMAZING, WONDERFUL NEWS was that my results were negative and scans showed that I was seemingly clear of the disease. However, I remember having been given this news once before. Therefore, I knew nothing was ever that easy and then came the bad news! Both specialists now suggested that I receive radiotherapy for a further four weeks on a daily basis to specifically target the sacrum, which is my tailbone. They felt that it was the best option, to ensure as best they could that the Lymphoma didn't return.

I couldn't believe it! I couldn't grasp that this horrible experience was to be extended, yet again! I knew if I didn't go through with it, my cancer had a much higher possibility of returning. Then, if it did return I would have to go through the entire chemo process yet again. Another new chemo treatment program would make the treatments I'd already undergone seem like a picnic, with the added probability of bone marrow transplants. I had just two weeks to decide.

CHAPTER 13

Unreal Dreams

Under Pressure

The next couple of weeks was a roller-coaster journey as I experienced a gamut of emotions from joy and rapture to annoyance and despair. Joyous, that I had finally finished my treatment and it was a surreal feeling. Those seemingly endless days of waking up and not knowing how the rest of my life was going to pan out, were now about to end. Just thinking about it brought tears to my eyes.

Of course my emotional and psychological self still had to recover and hopefully with time return to my former 'happy-go-lucky' state. I reasoned that once someone had been through such an ordeal, usually they became a better person possibly through growing a more grateful heart and viewing the world as a lucky second attempt to enjoy life. There were days when I would bounce around to tunes on the radio like "Rock your Body" by Justin Timberlake and "Get it Together" by India Arie.

However, annoyance and frustration frequently accompanied my daily mood swings. For anyone who has ever watched the musical movie "The Wizard of Oz", you would know that the tin-man had difficulty walking. Well, that was me, not only in walking but in kneeling, squatting and bending down, washing and drying my feet, putting on and taking my socks off, putting on and taking my shoes off and even tying my shoe laces.

Both my lower back and hips were almost paralysed. When I shared this with my haematologist, she said it could be due to the medication I had been prescribed. Apparently the Prednisone I'd been taking for several months may have masked inflammatory pains in my joints. Other medical professionals said that Prednisone can cause the joints to weaken and stiffen when taken over a sustained period.

My oncologist commented that my body had been through a great deal over the last few years and would take some time to recover. I honestly felt I had aged 20 years within the few months of the chemo treatment, but his best advice was for me to remain a patient patient... haha!

Another health professional commented that I was in relatively good shape for a person in their mid-forties. Even though I knew he was trying to pump me up I wasn't encouraged, I nevertheless appreciated the effort. All I really wanted was to be able to perform the same daily routines I'd always done, just as I did last year and the year before. I also felt perplexed that I still had to endure more physical suffering, emotional and mental anguish due to the imminent radiotherapy treatment.

I can't remember if I'd mentioned this earlier, but within just a few hours my body always started to respond in a negative way to whatever medication or antibiotic I ever took. My symptoms usually ranged from dizziness, fatigue, upset stomach, a cloudy mind, loss of appetite through too much pain and onset of a very short temper. To experience radiotherapy again with all this emotional hardship at the forefront of my mind, became a serious downer and I felt totally discouraged.

Family, friends and acquaintances that heard or asked what stage I was in, repeated the same response over and over again. ''Well, you've come this far, now you have only four weeks of treatment to go'' They sounded like parrots, all of them!

I understood where they were coming from and that all they wanted was the best for me and my family, and to give me some form of encouragement. However, when a person feels they can no longer take pain, trauma, physical, mental and emotional torture, and that they are almost spiritually depleted, it becomes almost impossible to feel encouraged. My strong faith had been stretched and stretched and stretched some more. At this point perhaps its worthwhile pointing out some examples of just where my frame of mind was and how I doubted my ability to ever shake myself clear of this horrendous cancer.

Example 1. I dreamt I had just run a gruelling marathon, my muscles were aching and my lungs were close to collapsing. I was about to run into the home straight, when the judge at the finishing line rang the bell and ordered me to run another 10 laps around the stadium.

Example 2. Another constant thought was that I was on a hike in freezing mountainous terrain, with treacherous climatic conditions, suffering frostbite on my toes and fingers. However, after much effort in reaching the summit, I found out that I couldn't set camp until I had climbed the huge mountain on the horizon because that was where my tent and supplies were.

Example 3. My final haunting apparition was that I had been put in the boxing ring with Mike Tyson and luckily survived all the rounds. I was bruised and battered, I had a broken jaw and busted ribs. I could hardly hold my gloves up, then the referee announced that it was a draw, and we needed to have an immediate rematch to determine the winner tonight.

It might seem strange that such negative thoughts constantly came to me, but such are the emotional hurdles that accompany the physical pain of dealing with the likes of cancer.

> *Finally be strong in the Lord and in his mighty power. Put on the full armour of God so that you can take your stand against the devils schemes. For our struggle is not against flesh and blood, but against the rulers, against the authorities, against the powers of this dark world and against the spiritual forces of evil in the heavenly realms.*
>
> *Ephesians 6:10-13*

Anguish

After a great deal of anguish, I succumbed to the thinking of the great Napoleon when he said, "impossible is a word to be found only in the dictionary of fools". So once again, it was 'head down, bum up' and 'full speed ahead' as I threw in my full resolve to complete this journey and undertake the radiotherapy.

Just a week before the radiotherapy was to be administered, a meeting took place between the oncologists, the oncologist registrar and myself. We went through all the questions, concerns and possibilities of what to expect as well as the possible side-effects of radiotherapy. We also painstakingly went through the medication I was required to take and the times to take them. My appointments were to be every day for four weeks, Monday to Friday for a duration of 10 to 15 minutes at a time.

All I could think of was an Aunty of mine, who had been diagnosed with bowel cancer and was given radiotherapy to stem the advancing malignancy. Unfortunately for my auntie, the technicians slightly overcooked the dose of radiation and inadvertently destroyed all the bone tissue in her lower abdomen. It was an absolute disaster and she finally succumbed to a terribly painful death some months later.

But it was now full speed ahead for me. So after a meeting of not even a full hour, all my queries had been answered and all bases had been covered. Of course the doctors wanted a smooth, trouble-free treatment just as much as I did, but we all knew there were always risks with radiotherapy. In coming through this meeting I felt quite relieved in a strange sort of way, at how empathetic they were for me.

They also knew what had happened a couple of years previously, when I had my first bout with radiotherapy in 2010. I recall that on that occasion I was constantly sick, endured nausea every day, dropped approximately 10kg and sometimes entered the hospital absolutely refusing to undergo any treatment at all. The experience made me obstinate, miserable and I absolutely hated every day of radiotherapy.

Now three years later, here I was, sitting in the same hospital room, still making these life-changing decisions. Was this episode of my life ever going to end? At the end of my consultation with the specialist staff, I was due to be 'tattooed' as they call it. Tattooing is having markings drawn on your body according to dimensions set down by the oncologist.

I felt like singing... 'Here we go, here we go, here we go', a generic chant in the world of football sung in a jovial manner by supporters before, during and after matches. Except that I was not in any way in a jovial mood. At times like these, another old favourite song often came to mind called ''Changes'' by Tupac.

"That's just the way it is, things will never be the same, that's just the way it is."

I started my treatment the following week. My appointments were booked for the late afternoon after work, between 4:30 and 5:15pm. This was so that if ever I felt unwell, I would have the rest of the evening to recuperate and would be able to sleep it off if necessary.

Surprisingly, but with God behind me, my next four weeks were strangely tolerable. I was able to work throughout the treatment without taking a single day off. I was also able to eat regularly even though my appetite was somewhat suppressed. I was even able to go to the gym for light workouts and on the whole I functioned on a daily basis as normal. I was surprisingly very, very happy with the way my radiotherapy treatment subsequently went. The following particular scripture always reassured me that we must overcome hardships to develop our own character.

Consider it pure joy my brothers whenever you face trials of many kinds, because you know that the testing of your faith develops perseverance.

Perseverance must finish its work so that you may be mature and complete, not lacking anything.

James 1:2-5

Giving Thanks

All the way through my perilous unknown journey, the company I work for had been extraordinarily supportive and showed a great deal of empathy towards me. In return, I pledged myself to be as supportive and helpful in return as their sympathy and encouragement of my situation was very much appreciated. My work classification was not administrative and I was not a member of the office staff. Neither did my job description include a managerial aspect, as I was the only person in my department. My financial contribution to the company was not one at the top of the ladder. I was definitely not one of the highest paid employees, quite the opposite.

My starting position was as a driver with catering knowledge and experience. Twelve months into the job I tore my rotator cuffs in both shoulders by repetitive heavy lifting in and out of the work vehicles. As a result of the injury I was placed on light duties and worked as a chef in a section that didn't require lifting and repetitive movement. This was until both my shoulders had fully recovered.

Yet, throughout my ordeal I always received phone calls from my employers to see how my progress was going. They were always very supportive and understanding, and assured me that my position remained safe until I returned to work. So, for them to continue their support throughout my cancer, was truly a magnificent gesture.

I had to trust God all the way through the treatment, all my family and friends prayed throughout as well. Despite the divine assistance I still had a few side-effects:

- Fatigue during and at the end of every day.
- Loss of appetite meaning I would have three smaller than usual meals per day.
- Stomach upset causing excess gas, which was quite embarrassing at times.
- Lower back, hip and hamstring joints and flexibility became even stiffer.
- My blood circulation required a boost.
- It took a much longer time to become and stay warm, due to kidney inefficiency.
- More supplements and vitamins had to be consumed to obtain a balance.

At this point I can recall thinking that if I were to be turned upside down and shaken, my body would have sounded like a box of 'Malteser's'. Generally, the oncology specialist and myself were both quite pleased with the ongoing treatment, and especially that I could attend my appointments without falling sick and requiring extra medication.

After the radiotherapy was completed, my follow-up appointment with the oncologist was agonisingly scheduled for a few months' time. I didn't have to wait for just days or weeks, but it was to be months away! WHY? My instructions during this time were to carefully monitor my recovery and take note of my health. However, there is a saying that "time waits for no man", which I thought applied to my present situation as I wasn't about to wait or put my life on hold yet again!

Trying to get back on the road to recovery was a peculiar feeling at first. The most appropriate scenario to describe my new lease on life was, like having been a prisoner who had served three years and was now being released back into the community. The weeks and months before the thought of being released was surreal with all the pre-activities going on in my head.

I had a multitude of projects to complete and achieve in a quest to satisfy my innermost self. My seemingly lost and empty self was unsure about where to start and I faced a maze of chores, duties and assignments, which lined up ready to be tackled and ticked off my to do list. Throughout my ordeal, people around us came to the rescue and our close friends Sam, Ginetta, Karen and Sherina cooked homemade meals for myself and my family on a regular basis.

My social calendar was now being booked up on a weekly basis to catch up with friends and relatives, and I chose cafes and restaurants to tantalise my taste buds. I felt I had now been authorized to become a part of normal everyday society. My pulse opened and closed like an accordion being pumped, and the world around me looked and felt so alive. My senses picked up on the mindless whining people who often became involved in idle chatter over such petty topics as the weather, the cost of petrol or how busy the traffic was.

For my particular goals to be achieved, a degree of planning had to be executed. Gratitude and being grateful for life's most simple and pure pleasures was also now a strong motivator, which played its part in my everyday thinking. Of course I had to tune into my body and listen for any warning signs. I had to get my internal system working efficiently again, and I knew if I pushed too soon, or too hard in a physical way, there would be consequences. All this took time, but I knew that everyday was a slow progressive step in the right direction.

My recovery was definitely sped up with the help of Dwayne, who was another one of Jude's cousins. Dwayne, who is married to Nic, was a regional manager for a major health supplement company. They've always been a great couple and were so kind to me throughout my lengthy treatment program. Nic was always happy to furnish me with advice and supplied me with good quality health supplements to take. This included products to improve the kidneys, liver, immune tolerance and phytogesics to alleviate joint issues and boost the metabolism. I'm sure these health supplements played an integral part in kick-starting my recovery.

CHAPTER 14

That's Life

I Can Breathe

Within a few days of my treatment coming to an end, our family's focus shifted from my health to my mother-in-law, Keriata's health. A few months previously, Keriata had developed pins and needles running down one of her arms, and after a few massages and doctors appointments it was still re-occurring. She was referred to a neurology specialist, who was very surprised that she was still able to walk and function as normal.

Unfortunately, a benign tumour was diagnosed situated at the back of the neck just inside her spinal cord, which had to be removed as soon as possible. The only way to treat this was to undergo emergency surgery. The consulting doctor was Charlie Teo, who is one of Australia's best known and most respected neuro-surgeons. It was a delicate procedure, but from the outset he was very confident he could perform the operation successfully.

Both our families were worried about the diagnosis, but relieved that the surgery could be undertaken quickly, and even more relieved that Dr. Teo was confident he could remove it. It was a very delicate nine-hour operation with a possibility of six to eighteen months in recuperation.

The operation was thankfully a success. Keriata stayed in hospital for a further four weeks and was then allowed home. Not only was her recovery fast, but her attitude to getting better was strong and confident. Her rehabilitation and physiotherapy was gradual however, and required a lot of patience. She is now doing very well and showers praise upon the support and medical staff, all of whom were involved with her operation and rehabilitation. Dr. Charlie Teo and his understudy both had a personal caring relationship with my mother-in-law and her husband, especially after the operation through follow-up calls and emails, which really meant a lot to them.

Having a completely different focus was good for me, it took my mind off my own problems and helped me to concentrate on my mother-in-law. I knew that by having a tight knit family, a local caring church, close friends and an intimate connection with God, Keriata would come through this health scare. In the end we were all surprised how smoothly everything turned out.

Unfortunately, that wasn't the end of our health concerns as my wife Jude was also going through her own physical challenges around this time. Her sleep was being constantly interrupted. The problem started in her neck, then spread to her shoulders and down her right arm. Over a period of three months she had to make regular visits to a physiotherapist, then a chiropractor. A specific program with a series of stretches was put in place for her to perform and practice plus a supportive pillow was purchased. Good advice from professional medical staff also helped. Jude's problems were definitely a result of her worrying, first over me and then her mother.

And I didn't come through my ordeal without problems either. My encounter with HL definitely left its mark on me. Physically I was left with huge bags under my eyes, with the left eye being much more noticeable. This wasn't apparent everyday, but enough for others to constantly remark or question if I'd had enough sleep.

I tried using eye gel plus rubbing cucumbers over my eyes for a couple of months. Then I became a little more realistic and made an appointment to see an eye specialist. After just ten minutes of the consultation, the specialist recommended that I should have a small operation to remove the excess fluid that was building up under my eyes. This unwanted fluid was apparently caused by the medications in combination with the treatment I had been through.

But I had to wait a further eight months as she was completely booked up. Because of what I'd been through, the eye specialist even gave me a reduction in the price, which was very much appreciated. So wait I did... and eight months later the operation was conducted. The simple surgery took a brief couple of hours with help from an eye anaesthetic. I was then sent home with an ice pack, eye drops and gel and my eyes returned to normal within days. The procedure was a complete success and even tidied up the eye a little, which was a bonus.

As if we weren't aware of it already, these events showed how vulnerable and how precious life is and made us appreciate what an amazing gift we all have in being alive!

Trust in the LORD with all your heart and lean not on your own understanding (5); in all your ways acknowledge him, and he will make your paths straight (6).

Proverbs 3:5-6

A Time To Reflect

For all the months prior to my recovery Jude had been my personal aide and carer, supporting me emotionally, physically, mentally and financially. A carer's role is to be there for everyone at anytime and Jude somehow kept the family together. Following is a shortlist of just some of the duties Jude performed in addition to her normal paid work:

- Learnt new things, e.g. cooking, paramedic, and masseuse.
- Kept life as normal as possible.
- Always had a sense of humour.
- Always asked if I needed help at any time.
- Knew the location of every emergency department in the area.

I put my ability to endure and recover so well down to Jude's personal sacrifice. A sacrifice is the giving up of something that is valued or forsaking something regarded as being important or worthy. Jude sacrificed all of her time, her patience, tolerance and love. By laying our life down for God, life will be laid out for us. There is no freedom without sacrifice!

I believe when we become more of who God wants us to be, freedom will empower us to do great things. Then you will know the truth and the truth will set you free.

Mark 8:32-33

Now it was my turn to give back and invest in my wife's well-being. During the next couple of months our family was kept abnormally busy and we attended a number of events. We attended an evening at our friends Bill and Helen's home for dinner. Bill and Helen had also invited a few of their friends around as well including Bessie, Alison and Manny. This night was one of fantastic food, great company and riotous laughter... a kind of coming out party. Other events included a 21st birthday of my wife's cousin; our friend's 50th birthday; a Hillsong conference in Homebush, and another friend's birthday at her house.

There were also a seemingly endless round of appointments with various medical professionals. Then there was a lunch meeting for all people who had survived blood related cancers and their carers. This was very enlightening and helpful to me personally as a way of saying thank you. Jude and I started Yoga classes together, which helped a lot with our flexibility, breathing and stress relief, and definitely aided us in getting a good night's sleep for a change.

In The Clear?

I had to undergo another PET scan prior to the final round of meetings, which were not scheduled until four months after I had completed all treatments. Eventually however, I was called in for what I hoped was to be 'the final meetings' with the haematologist, and another meeting with the oncologist. It all took time... a lot of time! But here I was about to receive the results, the news, the icing on the cake, the proof of the pudding... the real deal!

Dr. Susan didn't beat about the bush.

"Joseph, we've got the results and I'd like to report to you that we can no longer see any growth in your body. There is something there, but we honestly believe that it is debris from your treatment. Nothing is growing and we are happy with the result. You are now in remission". All this was said with a wry smile on her face.

How I felt at this point, with such great news was just pure relief! Yes... the medical staff all agreed that my results now showed no signs of the cancer. Yes... I was totally and overwhelmingly relieved that this infliction had been eradicated. And yes... the treatments were also all done. But unlike the Hollywood movies, sadly, that wasn't the end of it. Dr. Susan continued...

"Unfortunately, while I don't think it will happen, as your consulting doctor it is my duty to inform you that there is always a possibility that the cancer may at some time return. Therefore, for the foreseeable future, I would like you keep in touch with me and return to the hospital for blood tests every four months or so".

Of course I was relieved, but to be completely honest I also had mixed feelings about the fact that I had to return to the hospital, which definitely left me feeling somewhat confused.

So... yes, the cancer had a possibility of returning. And... I still had to come back to the hospital every few months for blood tests. After days, weeks, months of pain, torment, nausea and worry, I asked myself when will all the tests and monitoring end? Once you have had cancer, was it the inevitable plan to be tested for the rest of your life? "Phew" was my overwhelming thought, but I also felt sort of let down that there was no clear-cut outcome.

That day there were no backflips or somersaults, no punching the air to show how happy I was, but like diving into a pool or downing a cold beer on a hot day, I definitely felt relief... ahhhh! Although absolutely elated, I was nevertheless guarded about the future and this same approach was the very same manner I used to inform my family and friends of the outcome.

Life is a journey with lots of bumps and bruises along the way. I've come to discover that it's all about attitude and our ability to persist and persevere. I guess we don't really ever know 100% if we are or will be 100% for the rest of our lives, but I live 100% in the belief that the deadly disease which made me sick all that time has gone, never to be seen again. All I had to do now, was ensure that stress was eradicated from my life and that I kept myself fit and healthy.

On my personal journey there were many days when I faced the prospect of eternity. The experience taught me that when doubt, fear and negativity comes into our lives, it has a knock-on effect on our well-being and paralyses the future. God in all his greatness has provided us with a tapestry of grace and love, which in turn grants us freedom and endless opportunity. Thankfully, life was now slowly returning to normal again. I was immensely enjoying getting back to basics with the tiniest of things like appreciating a simple drink of water.

You must know by now that I have a love of music. About now

I was listening to an old favourite of mine called "Hyper Paradise," the Flume remix by Hermitude, which always made me get up and dance! I just love that tune and listened to it over and over on my headphones! Music definitely kept me going especially when I was down and felt hopeless about my situation.

Even though my immune system is not as strong as it used to be, and the joints in my hips, knees and shoulders are weakened with arthritis, I feel wonderful about life and my place in it. My gym sessions are now consistent with my diet and nutritional needs. My current workplace involves catering and looking after patients who are treated by very successful doctors and surgeons in a supportive and caring private hospital.

Jude, Tahlia and I have since moved to a cosy apartment in Kensington, which is convenient and practical for myself and my family's needs. We are part of an inspiring International Hillsong Church, led by visionaries Brian and Bobbie Houston, who are full of love for God and their people. We regularly see and hear the thousands of lives this church impacts upon, mentors and assists its members on a daily basis, and we live just ten minutes away from our City Campus. We serve every two weeks in the Welcome Lounge, and under great service Pastors Fior and Pina, who are so inspiring, we assist amongst a great team of volunteer's eager to please God.

If you looked at me now, you wouldn't be able to tell what I had been through the last couple of years. I've realised that such random misfortunes can happen to anyone at anytime. Sometimes the events and suffering we go through can change or distort our perception of life. We don't know why these things happen, we just have to get on with it as best we can under the circumstances. But what I do know is this:

"All things work together for good for those who know the Lord"

Romans 8:13.

We are all on a journey, whether you are pursuing your dreams, looking for adventure or simply at a cross-road and unsure of the next step. The key is to never give up, believe and have faith, and we don't have to do it alone.

> *Because he loves me says the Lord, I will rescue him*
> *I will protect he that acknowledges my name*
> *Call upon me and I will answer him*
> *I will be with him in trouble,*
> *I will deliver him and honour him*
> *With long life will I satisfy him*
> *And show him my salvation*
>
> *Psalm a1:14-16*

This was my journey into the unknown.

Thank You

I need to thank my wife Jude, whose love, patience and tolerance was always unlimited, along with the rest of my family here in Australia, England and New Zealand. They know me the best, their love and encouragement carried me through the emotional peaks and valleys. I would also like to acknowledge my close friends who made our accommodation and everyday living expenses easier to manage. They stood shoulder to shoulder with me and my family through the everyday battles we often had and spoke wisdom when it was most needed.

I am most particularly grateful to my consulting medical specialists, in particular Dr. Susan MacCallum, and the staff who work in the Oncology Unit at the Prince of Wales Hospital in Randwick, NSW. Many thanks too are due to all my Christian brothers and sisters who donated their time, prayers, finances and Godly experience, which delivered unto me a deep spiritual and inner strength.

I am grateful to all my work peers and colleagues who were so courteous to me in the workplace, and whose empathy and flexibility allowed me to rest when I was physically exhausted. I also wish to thank those persons (too many to acknowledge) that helped my family and I throughout my struggle. Sincere thanks too for those that helped edit my story. I must also thank my publisher, Dr. Tracy Rockwell of Pegasus Publishing whose experience, insight and perseverance enabled me to turn my scratchy diary into this book.

Finally I would like to thank you the readers, whose families, friends and neighbours prompted me to be vocal about an everyday illness no one dares to talk about openly. Be positive, life is amazing!

Joseph

Lightning Source UK Ltd.
Milton Keynes UK
UKHW020625090519
342383UK00014B/1390/P

9 780994 201492